GLOSSARY OF VETERINARY TERMS
FRENCH-ENGLISH AND ENGLISH-FRENCH
BY

GLOSSAIRE DES TERMES VÉTÉRINAIRES
FRANÇAIS-ANGLAIS ET ANGLAIS-FRANÇAIS
PAR

SUSAN KIRKHAM

HADLEY PAGER INFO

First Edition 2006

ISBN 1-872739-17-2
(978-1-872739-17-5)

Printed and bound in England by Antony Rowe Ltd.,
Chippenham

HADLEY PAGER INFO
Leatherhead, Surrey, England

FOREWORD

In preparing the Glossary of Veterinary Terms I have consulted a wide range of veterinary literature both in French and in English. I am also greatly indebted to Alan Lindsey for providing the results of a preliminary study of French veterinary terms which has helped to lighten my task.

This Glossary will be of value to pet owners taking their pets to France on holiday or those permanently living in France with pets, when they wish to consult a vet. It is assumed that the user of this Glossary will have a basic knowledge of French, however some general notes have been included to give additional help. Conversely this Glossary will assist French pet owners when visiting the United Kingdom.

The Pet Passport scheme is now available to control the movement of domestic pets between the UK and the Continent and some details of these regulations are included here. However it should be emphasised that these regulations are subject to revision at any time and it is the responsibility of the traveller to conform to the most recent regulations. The website addresses of DEFRA and of the British Embassy in France have been included to permit a check of the most recent amendments.

Finally I should also like to thank Alan Lindsey again for providing the Lists of Cat, Dog and Horse Breeds included as an appendix. So that the glossary can be improved in future editions I would greatly appreciate readers reporting any errors of omission or commission that they might notice.

S. K.

Abbreviations Used

abb	abbreviation	agric	agricultural
adj	adjective		
f	feminine	™	Trade Mark or
	noun		Name
m	masculine		
	noun		
pl	plural form		

It should be noted that the definitions given in this dictionary have no legal or statutory basis. Entered words which the author has reason to believe are registered trade names or marks, or which have been used as trade names or marks are indicated by the symbol ™. However, the presence or absence of such a symbol should not be regarded as affecting the legal status of any trade mark or name.

CONTENTS

ENGLISH-FRENCH

VISIT TO THE VET

**USEFUL WORDS AND PHRASES WHEN SPEAKING TO
THE VET ON THE TELEPHONE OR IN THE SURGERY**
(See general notes at end of this section, pages 15-17)

My (cat, dog, horse, pony, puppy etc) is	Mon* (chat, chien, cheval, poney, chiot, etc) est [* ma for female animals]
Unwell	Souffrant,-e
Ill	Malade
Injured	Blessé
It is serious	C'est grave
It is urgent	C'est urgent
It isn't urgent	Ce n'est pas urgent
I'd like an appointment, please	Je voudrais un rendez-vous, s'il vous plaît
As soon as possible	Aussitôt que possible
It is essential that....	Il faut absolument que....
What is the telephone number of....?	Qu'est-ce que le numéro de téléphone de....?
Where is...?	Où se trouve...?
A vet	Un vétérinaire
Yes	Oui
No	Non
Please	S'il vous plaît
Thank you	Merci
Good morning	Bonjour
Good evening	Bonsoir
Goodbye	Au revoir
Excuse me	Pardon

9

Sorry	Je m'excuse/je suis désolé,-e
Sir	Monsieur
Madam	Madame
Necessary	Nécessaire
Later	Plus tard
Next week	La semaine prochaine
Last week	La semaine dernière
Last night	Hier soir
Form	La feuille
Alternative medicine	Les médecines douces
Surgery (place)	Le cabinet
Surgery (operation)	La chirurgie
Chemist /pharmacy	La pharmacie
Town centre	Centre ville
Free (no cost)	Gratuit
Closed	Fermé
Open	Ouvert
No smoking	Défense de fumer
Good	Bon, bonne
Well	Bien
Almost	Presque
Early	Tôt
Earlier	Plus tôt
Late	Tard
Late (to be)	En retard (être)
Later	Plus tard

AT THE VET'S SURGERY

USEFUL EXPRESSIONS	PHRASES UTILES
I have an appointment with Mr. X, the vet	J'ai un rendez-vous avec Monsieur X, le vétérinaire
At half-past four	À seize heures et demie
Do you speak English ?	Parlez-vous anglais?
Is there anyone here who speaks English ?	Est-ce qu'il y a quelqu'un qui parle anglais?
Please speak more slowly	Parlez plus lentement s'il vous plaît
I don't understand	Je ne comprends pas
What does that mean ?	Qu'est-ce que ça veut dire ?
What does that word mean ?	Qu'est-ce que ce mot veut dire?
How much is that ?	C'est combien ?
How would you like to pay ?	Comment voudriez-vous régler?
I'd like to pay in cash/by credit card/by cheque	Je voudrais régler en espèces/par carte bancaire/par chèque
Can I help you ?	Puis-je vous aider ?
Can you help me?	Est-ce que vous pouvez m'aider?
What is the matter ?	Qu'est-ce qui a ?
I have a problem with....	J'ai un problème avec....
I'd like some information/advice about....	Je voudrais des renseignements/des conseils sur....
Can you come back tomorrow/Monday/next week ?	Vous pouvez revenir demain/lundi/la semaine prochaine?

I need…	Il me faut…/J'ai besoin de…
What's happening ?	Qu'est-ce que se passe ?
I don't know	Je ne sais pas
Would you write it down	L'inscrivez, s'il vous plaît
What is his/her name?	Comment s'appelle-t-il/elle?
His/her name is….	Il/elle s'appelle….
What is your name?	Comment vous appelez-vous?
My name is….	Je m'appelle….
How is that written?	Comment ça s'inscrit?
At what time?	A quelle heure?
Put him/her here/there	Posez-le/la par ici/là
On the table	Sur la table
On the floor	Sur le plancher
Hold him/her here	Tenez-le/la ici
Hold him/her still	Tenez-le/la tranquille
When did you first notice?	Vous l'avez remarqué quand?
She's/he's eating very little	Elle/il ne mange que peu
I've tried to make him/her eat	J'ai essayé de le/la faire manger
She/he is constipated	Elle/il est constipé/e
She/he has diarrhoea	Elle/il a la diarrhée
She/he is drinking a lot	Elle/il boit beaucoup
She/he isn't drinking much	Elle/il ne boit que peu
I think she/he is in pain	Je crois que qu'elle/il souffre
The last time, my vet…	La dernière fois, le vétérinaire…
I have changed his/her food recently	Je viens de changer son alimentation
You must change his/her food	Il lui faut un changement d'alimentation
Have there been any changes at home?	Est ce qu'il y a quelque chose de différent chez vous?
It happened quickly/slowly	C'est arrivé vite/lentement

She/he got worse quickly/ slowly	Son état s'est aggravé vite/ lentement
I haven't noticed anything	Je n'ai rien remarqué
You must follow the treatment for … days	Il faut suivre le traitement pendant … jours
I am going back to the UK	Je rentre au Royaume-Uni
I am going back to France	Je rentre en France
I need an EU Pet's Passport	Il me faut un passeport EU pour mon animal de compagnie
Can you give me one?	Pouvez-vous m'en délivrer un ?
A blood sample was taken on …	On a fait une prise de sang le …
Do you need my Pet's Passport?	Est-ce qu'il vous faut le passeport de mon animal de compagnie ?
My vet issued it	C'était délivré par mon vétérinaire
Can you give the necessary treatment against ticks and tapeworms?	Pouvez-vous traiter mon animal contre les tiques et les ténias, comme c'est nécessaire ?
I need an official certificate of treatment	J'ai besoin d'un certificat officiel, prouvant le traitement
My dog/cat has been vaccinated against rabies	Mon chien/chat a été vacciné contre la rage
Does my dog/cat need to be vaccinated against rabies?	Est-ce qu'il faut vacciner mon chien/chat contre la rage ?
I do not live in France so my animal does not need to be tattooed	Je ne suis pas résident en France donc il ne faut pas que mon animal soit tatoué

Check its teeth	Faire vérifier ses dents
My pet has a problem with its foreleg/hindleg	Mon animal a un problème avec la jambe antérieure/postérieure
My pet has difficulty standing up	C'est difficile pour mon animal de se lever
My pet has a lump on its leg/stomach/side/head	Mon animal a un grosseur sur la jambe/le ventre/le flanc/la tête
My pet has a sore patch	Mon animal a une plaie
My pet keeps chewing at ..	Mon animal continue à se mordiller le/la..
To be taken …times a day	À prendre … fois par jour
To be taken on an empty stomach	À prendre à jeun
Do not exceed the prescribed dose	Ne pas dépasser la dose prescrite

SOME GENERAL NOTES ON THE FRENCH LANGUAGE

The verbs you will need to use in conversation most often are
ÊTRE and **AVOIR.**

To be	Être	To have	Avoir
I am	Je suis	I have	J'ai
You are (familiar)	Tu es	You are (familiar)	Tu as
He is	Il est	He has	Il a
She is	Elle est	She has	Elle a
We are	Nous sommes	We have	Nous avons
You are	Vous êtes	You have	Vous avez
They are	Ils/elles sont	They have	Ils/elles ont

A useful phrase when you need something is: -

Je voudrais   I'd like

e.g. Je voudrais un rendez-vous   I'd like an appointment

USEFUL NUMBERS FOR TIME

One	Un, une	Seventeen	Dix-sept
Two	Deux	Eighteen	Dix-huit
Three	Trois	Nineteen	Dix-neuf
Four	Quatre	Twenty	Vingt
Five	Cinq	Twenty-one	Vingt-et-un
Six	Six	Twenty-two	Vingt-deux
Seven	Sept	Twenty-three	Vingt-trois
Eight	Huit	Twenty-four	Vingt-quatre
Nine	Neuf	Twenty-five	Vingt-cinq
Ten	Dix	Thirty	Trente
Eleven	Onze	Thirty-five	Trente-cinq
Twelve	Douze	Forty	Quarante
Thirteen	Treize	Forty-five	Quarante-cinq
Fourteen	Quatorze	Fifty	Cinquante
Fifteen	Quinze	Fifty-five	Cinquante-cinq
Sixteen	Seize		

TIME

Most people in France use the 24 hour clock, thus an appointment in the afternoon would be at 16 hours (**seize heures**) and not 4 p.m. For times past or to the hour it is expressed by the hour plus the number e.g.16.10, (**seize heures dix**); 17.45, (**dix-sept heures quarante-cinq**).

DAYS and MONTHS

DAYS	LES JOURS
Monday	lundi
Tuesday	mardi
Wednesday	mercredi
Thursday	jeudi
Friday	vendredi
Saturday	samedi
Sunday	dimanche

MONTHS	LES MOIS
January	janvier
February	fevrier
March	mars
April	avril
May	mai
June	juin
July	juillet
August	août
September	septembre
October	octobre
November	novembre
December	decembre

DATES

1st of March = le premier mars
Tuesday, 27th January = mardi, le vingt-sept janvier
At the beginning/end of September = au debut/à la fin du mois de septembre
Tomorrow morning = demain matin
Tomorrow afternoon = demain après-midi

PETS' PASSPORTS

The information given here is a general summary of the main requirements for Pet's Passports and was accurate at the time of publication. For further and updated information consult the defra website for information in English:- **www.defra.gov.uk**
And the British Embassy in France website for information in French:- **www.amb-grandebretagne.fr**

(Go to VISAS, IMPORTATIONS then Programme de Voyage des Animaux de Compagnie)

Since 3rd July 2004, dogs, cats, ferrets, pet rabbits, rodents and other pets travelling between EU and associated countries are required to travel with a European pet's passport. An existing Pet Travel Scheme (PETS) certificate can be used until its expiration date.

N.B. Guide dogs and similar working dogs are not exempt from the legislation.

The requirement for rabies treatment applies to all dogs, cats and ferrets.

Travelling from the United Kingdom to France
The animal
- Must travel on an approved route. Not all carriers will accept every type of animal.
- Must be at least 3 months old.
- Must be identifiable by a microchip implanted under the skin. The microchip must conform to ISO standards.
- Must have been vaccinated against rabies and have a valid certificate for this.

- Must have had a blood test to prove the vaccination was successful and have a certificate to show this.
- Must have been treated against ticks and tapeworms. The treatment must have been carried out by a vet. Anti-parasite treatment is not required for pets returning to France.
- Must be accompanied by a certificate of identity and a declaration that it has not been outside the participating countries during the previous 6 months.

The French authorities will accept all valid PETS certificates provided that they are written in both French and English. Certificates issued by the French authorities are bilingual.

Travelling from France to the United Kingdom
The animal
- Must travel on an approved route. Not all carriers will accept every type of animal. Pets cannot be brought into the UK from private planes and boats.
- Must be at least 3 months old.
- Must be identifiable by a microchip implanted under the skin. Tattooing alone is not accepted. The microchip must conform to ISO standards.
- Must have been vaccinated against rabies and have a valid certificate for this.
- Must have had a blood test to prove the vaccination was successful and have a certificate to show this. The animal cannot enter the UK until 6 months after a successful blood test.
- Must have been treated against ticks and tapeworms. The treatment must have been carried out by a vet. The timing

for this is critical i.e. between 24 to 48 hours prior to entry into the UK.
- Must be accompanied by a certificate of identity and a declaration that it has not been outside the participating countries during the previous 6 months.

Horses

European legislation requires all horses, ponies and donkeys to have a passport, even if the animal is not travelling abroad.
Veterinary certificates are not passports.
Bilingual documentation is available.

The defra website has full details:-
   www.defra.gov.uk/rural/horses

FRANÇAIS-ANGLAIS

AU CABINET DU VÉTÉRINAIRE

MOTS ET EXPRESSIONS UTILES QUAND VOUS ÊTES AU TELEPHONE OU AU CABINET DU VÉTÉRINAIRE
(Voir les notes générales à la fin de cette section, p. 26-28)

Mon* (chat, chien, cheval, poney, chiot, etc) est [* ma pour les animaux femelles]	My (cat, dog, horse, pony, puppy, etc) is
Souffrant,-e	Unwell
Malade	Ill
Blessé,-e	Injured
C'est grave	It is serious
C'est urgent	It is urgent
Ce n'est pas urgent	It isn't urgent
Je voudrais un rendez-vous, s'il vous plaît	I'd like an appointment, please
Aussitôt que possible	As soon as possible
Il faut absolument que….	It is essential that….
Qu'est-ce que le numéro de téléphone de….?	What is the telephone number of….?
Où se trouve…?	Where is…?
Un vétérinaire	A vet
Oui	Yes
Non	No
S'il vous plaît	Please
Merci	Thank you
Bonjour	Good morning
Bonsoir	Good evening
Au revoir	Goodbye
Pardon	Excuse me

21

Je m'excuse/je suis désolé,-e	Sorry
Monsieur	Sir
Madame	Madam
Nécessaire	Necessary
Aujourd'hui	Today
Demain	Tomorrow
Plus tard	Later
La semaine prochaine	Next week
La semaine dernière	Last week
Hier soir	Last night
Le rendez-vous	Appointment
La feuille	Form
Les médecines douces	Alternative medicine
Le cabinet	Surgery (place)
La chirurgie	Surgery (operation)
La pharmacie	Chemist /pharmacy
Centre ville	Town centre
Gratuit	Free (no cost)
Fermé	Closed
Ouvert	Open
Défense de fumer	No smoking
Bon/bonne	Good
Bien	Well
Presque	Almost
Tôt	Early
Plus tôt	Earlier
Tard	Late
En retard (être)	Late (to be)
Plus tard	Later

AU CABINET DU VÉTÉRINAIRE

PHRASES UTILES

USEFUL EXPRESSIONS

J'ai un rendez-vous avec Monsieur X, le vétérinaire	I have an appointment with Mr. X, the vet
À quatre heures et demie	At half past four
Parlez-vous français?	Do you speak French ?
Est-ce qu'il y a quelqu'un qui parle français?	Is there anyone here who speaks French ?
Parlez plus lentement s'il vous plaît	Please speak more slowly
Je ne comprends pas	I don't understand
Qu'est-ce que ça veut dire ?	What does that mean ?
Qu'est-ce que ce mot veut dire?	What does that word mean ?
C'est combien ?	How much is that ?
Comment voudriez-vous régler?	How would you like to pay ?
Je voudrais régler en espèces/par carte bancaire/par chèque	I'd like to pay in cash/by credit card/by cheque
Puis-je vous aider ?	Can I help you ?
Est-ce que vous pouvez m'aider?	Can you help me?
Qu'est-ce qui a ?	What is the matter ?
J'ai un problème avec….	I have a problem with….
Je voudrais des renseignements/ des conseils sur….	I'd like some information/advice about….
Vous pouvez revenir demain/lundi/la semaine prochaine?	Can you come back tomorrow/Monday/next week ?
Il me faut…/J'ai besoin de…	I need…
Qu'est-ce que se passe ?	What's happening ?
Je ne sais pas	I don't know
L'inscrivez, s'il vous plaît	Would you write it down

Comment s'appelle-t-il/elle?	What is his/her name?
Il/elle s'appelle….	His/her name is….
Comment vous appelez-vous?	What is your name?
Je m'appelle….	My name is….
Comment ça s'inscrit?	How is that written?
A quelle heure?	At what time?
Posez-le/la par ici/là	Put him/her here/there
Sur la table	On the table
Sur le plancher	On the floor
Tenez-le/la ici	Hold him/her here
Tenez-le/la tranquille	Hold him/her still
Vous l'avez remarqué quand?	When did you first notice?
Elle/il ne mange que peu	She's/he's eating very little
J'ai essayé de le/la faire manger	I've tried to make him/her eat
Elle/il est constipé/e	She/he is constipated
Elle/il a la diarrhée	She/he has diarrhoea
Elle/il boit beaucoup	She/he is drinking a lot
Elle/il ne boit que peu	She/he isn't drinking much
Je crois que qu'elle/il souffre	I think she/he is in pain
La dernière fois, le vétérinaire…	The last time, my vet…
Je viens de changer son alimentation	I have changed his/her food recently
Il lui faut un changement d'alimentation	You must change his/her food
Est ce qu'il y a quelque chose de différent chez vous?	Have there been any changes at home?
C'est arrivé vite/lentement	It happened quickly/slowly
Son état s'est aggravé vite/lentement	She/he got worse quickly/slowly
Je n'ai rien remarqué	I haven't noticed anything
Je rentre au Royaume-Uni	I am going back to the UK
Je rentre en France	I am going back to France
Il me faut un passeport EU pour	I need an EU Pet's Passport

mon animal de compagnie
Pouvez-vous m'en délivrer un ?

Can you give me one?

On a fait une prise de sang le …

A blood sample was taken on …

Est-ce qu'il vous faut le passeport de mon animal de compagnie ?

Do you need my Pet's Passport?

C'était délivré par mon vétérinaire

My vet issued it

Pouvez-vous traiter mon animal contre les tiques et les ténias, comme c'est nécessaire ?

Can you give the necessary treatment against ticks and tapeworms?

J'ai besoin d'un certificat officiel, prouvant le traitement

I need an official certificate of treatment

Mon chien/chat a été vacciné contre la rage

My dog/cat has been vaccinated against rabies

Est-ce qu'il faut vacciner mon chien/chat contre la rage ?

Does my dog/cat need to be vaccinated against rabies?

Je ne suis pas résident en France donc il ne faut pas que mon animal soit tatoué

I do not live in France so my animal does not need to be tattooed

Faire vérifier ses dents

Check its teeth

Mon animal a un problème avec la jambe antérieure/ postérieure

My pet has a problem with its foreleg/hindleg

C'est difficile pour mon animal de se lever

My pet has difficulty standing up

Mon animal a un grosseur sur la jambe/le ventre/le flanc/la tête

My pet has a lump on its leg/stomach/side/head

Mon animal a une plaie

My pet has a sore patch

Mon animal continue à se mordiller le/la..

My pet keeps chewing at ..

Il faut suivre le traitement pendant … jours

You must follow the treatment for … days

À prendre … fois par jour

To be taken …times a day

À prendre à jeun		To be taken on an empty stomach	
Ne pas dépasser la dose prescrite		Do not exceed the prescribed dose	

NOTES GÉNÉRALES SUR LA LANGUE ANGLAIS

Les verbes qu'il vous faudra le plus souvent sont **TO BE** and **TO HAVE**

Être	To be	Avoir	To have
Je suis	I am	J'ai	I have
Tu es	You are (familiar)	Tu as	You are (familiar)
Il est	He is	Il a	He has
Elle est	She is	Elle a	She has
Nous sommes	We are	Nous avons	We have
Vous êtes	You are	Vous avez	You have
Ils/elles sont	They are	Ils/elles ont	They have

Quand il vous faut quelque chose, une phrase utile est :-
I'd like   Je voudrais
e.g. I'd like an appointment   Je voudrais un rendez-vous

DES NUMÉROS UTILES POUR L'HEURE

Un, une	One	Dix-sept	Seventeen
Deux	Two	Dix-huit	Eighteen
Trois	Three	Dix-neuf	Nineteen
Quatre	Four	Vingt	Twenty
Cinq	Five	Vingt-et-un	Twenty-one
Six	Six	Vingt-deux	Twenty-two
Sept	Seven	Vingt-trois	Twenty-three
Huit	Eight	Vingt-quatre	Twenty-four
Neuf	Nine	Vingt-cinq	Twenty-five
Dix	Ten	Trente	Thirty
Onze	Eleven	Trente-cinq	Thirty-five
Douze	Twelve	Quarante	Forty
Treize	Thirteen	Quarante-cinq	Forty-five
Quatorze	Fourteen	Cinquante	Fifty
Quinze	Fifteen	Cinquante-cinq	Fifty-five
Seize	Sixteen		

L'HEURE

En le Royaume-Uni, le plupart des gens n'utilise que les numéros 1 à 12 pour dire l'heure. Donc il faut préciser, par exemple, si c'est six heures du matin ou de soir.

LES JOURS ET LES MOIS

LES JOURS	DAYS
lundi	Monday
mardi	Tuesday
mercredi	Wednesday
jeudi	Thursday
vendredi	Friday
samedi	Saturday
dimanche	Sunday

LES MOIS	MONTHS
janvier	January
fevrier	February
mars	March
avril	April
mai	May
juin	June
juillet	July
août	August
septembre	September
octobre	October
novembre	November
decembre	December

DATES

le premier mars = 1st of March
mardi, le vingt-sept janvier = Tuesday, 27th January
au debut/à la fin du mois de septembre = at the beginning/end of
September
demain matin = tomorrow morning
demain après-midi = tomorrow afternoon

PROGRAMME DE VOYAGE DES ANIMAUX DE COMPAGNIE (PVAC)

Les renseignements ci-dessous offrent un résumé des conditions générales pour le PVAC. Ils étaient précisù au moment de publication. Pour se mettre au courant consulter :-
www.defra.gov.uk pour des renseignements en anglais et pour des renseignements en français.
www.amb-grandebretagne.gov.uk

(visiter VISAS, IMPORTATIONS puis Programme de Voyage des Animaux de Compagnie)

Depuis 3 juillet 2004 tout animal de compagnie qui voyage en les pays soussignés au PVAC doit remplir les conditions du PVAC. Un certificat PETS est encore valable jusqu'au date d'expiration.

Les conditions du PVAC doivent être remplies même par les chiens d'aveugle et les autres chiens d'assistance.

La vaccination contre la rage est obligatoire pour tous les chiens, chats et furets.

Entrée en France de Royaume-Uni
L'animal
- Doit être acheminé suivant un itinéraire autorisé. Il faut aussi s'assurer que la compagnie acceptera l'animal.
- Doit être âgé d'au moins de 3 mois.
- Doit être identifié par une micropuce implantée sous la peau. La micropuce doit conformer aux normes de l'ISO.
- Doit être vacciné contre la rage.
- Doit avoir subi un test sérologique.

- Doit avoir subi un traitement contre les tiques et l'échinococcose, fait par un vétérinaire. Le traitement n'est pas exigé pour rentrer en France.
- Doit être accompagné d'un certificat sanitaire attestant que l'animal a rempli les conditions d'identification et de vaccination antirabique, d'un certificat de traitement antiparasitaire et d'une déclaration de résidence attestant que l'animal n'a pas quitté les pays du PVAC pendant les six mois précédents.

Les autorités françaises ont convenu d'accepter tous certificats PETS encore valables à condition que les certificats soient bilingues. Les certificats délivrés par les autorités françaises sont bilingues.

Entrée au Royaume-Uni de France
L'animal
- Doit être acheminé suivant un itinéraire autorisé. Il faut aussi s'assurer que la compagnie acceptera l'animal. Un animal de compagnie ne peut pas entrer au Royaume-Uni ni d'un avion privé ni d'un bateau privé.
- Doit être âgé d'au moins de 3 mois.
- Doit être identifiée par une micropuce implantée sous la peau. La micropuce doit conformer aux normes de l'ISO. Le tatouage n'est pas accepté par les autorités britanniques.
- Doit être vacciné contre la rage.
- Doit avoir subi un test sérologique. L'animal ne peut pas entrer au Royaume-Uni avant 6 mois après le test sérologique.

- Doit avoir subi un traitement contre les tiques et
  l'échinococcose, fait par un vétérinaire. Le traitement doit
  être fait entre 24 et 48 heures avant l'entrée au Royaume-
  Uni .Doit être accompagné d'un certificat sanitaire
  attestant que l'animal a rempli les conditions
  d'identification et de vaccination antirabique, d'un
  certificat de traitement antiparasitaire et d'une déclaration
  de résidence attestant que l'animal n'a pas quitté les pays
  soussignés au PVAC pendant les six mois précédents.

Chevaux
La loi européenne demande que chaque cheval, poney, âne etc
doive être muni d'un passeport, même si l'animal ne quitte pas
son pays. Les certificats vétérinaires ne sont pas suffisants.
Il existe des passeports bilingues.
Le site defra offre plus de renseignements :-
www.defra.gov.uk:rural/horses.

GLOSSARY

ENGLISH-FRENCH

A

abandonning of the litter abandon *m* des jeunes
abatement (pain, etc) rémission *f*
abcess abcès *m*
abdomen abdomen *m*
abdominal abdominal,-e
abdominal aorta aorte *f* abdominale
abdominal cavity cavité *f* abdominale
abdominal swelling enflure *f* abdominale
abduction abduction *f*
aberrant aberrant,-e
aberration aberration *f*
abnormal position posture *f* anormale
abnormality défaut *m*
abortion avortement *m*
abrasion écorchure *f*; érosion *f*
absorbent absorbant,-e
absorbent cotton , cotton wool ouate *f* hydrophile
abstention from food jeûne *m*
achalasia achalasie *f*
accessory carpal bone os *m* accessoire du carpe
accident accident *m*
acetabulum acétabulum *m*
Achilles tendon tendon *m* d'Achille
acidosis acidose *f*
ascites ascite *f*
acne acné *f*
acne (spot) bouton *m* d'acné
acorns glands *mpl*
acquired immunity immunité *f* acquise
acquired immunity deficiency syndrome syndrome *m* immuno-déficitaire acquis
acromegalia; acromegaly acromégalie *f*

32

acuity, acuteness acuité *f*
acupuncture acupuncture *f*
acute aigu, aiguë
acute pulmonary oedema œdème *m* aigu du poumon
addiction addiction *f*
addiction dépendence *f*
Addison's disease maladie *f* d'Addison
adenitis adénite *f*
adenoma adénome *m*
adhesion adhérence *f*
adhesive bandage bande *f* adhésive
adhesive plaster pansement *m* adhésif
adhesive plaster sparadrap *m*
adipose tissue tissu *m* adipeux
adrenaline adrénaline *f*
adult adulte *m*
aelurostrangulus abstrusus infestation infestation *f*
    d'aelurostrangulus abstrusus
aetiology étiologie *f*
affect, to; reach, to atteindre
affected atteint,-e
affection affection *f*
afterbirth placenta *m*
aftercare post-cure *f*
after-effects séquelles *fpl*
agalactia agalactie *f*
age âge *m*
ageing vieillissement *m*
agglutinate, to agglutiner
agglutination agglutination *f*
agglutinin agglutinine *f*
aggressive agressif/agressive
aggressive behaviour comportement *m* agressif
ailment affectin *f*
airway voie *f* respiratoire
airway obstruction obstruction *f* de la voie respiratoire
albinism albinisme *m*
albino albinos
albumin albumine *f*
albuminuria albuminurie *f*

33

alcohol alcool *m*
alimentary canal tube *m* digestif
alkalosis alcalose *f*
allergen allergène *m*
allergic,to allergique à
allergy allergie *f*
all-purpose polyvalent,-e
alopecia alopécie *f*
alternative medicine médicine *f* douce
alula alula *m*
alveolitis of the lungs alvéolite *f* pulmonaire
amino acid acide *m* aminé
amniotic amniotique
amniotic fluid liquide *m* amniotique
amniotic sac poche *f* des eaux
amphetamine amphétamine *f*
ampulla ampoule *f*
amputation amputation *f*
amyloidosis amyloïdose *f*
anabolic steroid steroïde *m* anabolisant
anabolic steroid anabolisant *m*
anabolic steroid anabolisant *m* stéroïdien
anabolism anabolisme *m*
anaemia anémie *f*
anaemic anémique
anaerobic anérobique
anaesthesia anasthésie *f*
anaesthetic anesthésique *m*
anaesthetize, to anesthésier
anal adenomata circumanalomes *mpl*
anal glands glandes *fpl* anales
anal sphincter sphincter *m* anal
analgesic analgésique *m*
analgesic antalgique
analgesic calmant *m* analgésique
analysis analyse *f*
anaphylactic shock choc *m* anaphylactique
anaphylaxia anaphylaxie *f*
ancestry ascendance *f*
aneurism anévrisme *m*

angina angine *f* de poitrine
angioma angiome *m*
ankle cheville *f*
ankyloblepharon ankyloblépharon *m*
ankylostomiasis ankylostamiase *f*
anoestrus anœstrus *m*
anomaly anomalie *f*
anorexia anorexie *f*
anorexic anorexique
anoura anoure
anoxia anoxie *f*
anterior chamber of the eye chambre *f* antérieure de l'œil
anthelmintic antihelmintique *m*
anthrax charbon *m*
antibiotic antibiotique *m*
antibiotic ointment pommade *f* antibiotique
antibodies anticorps *mpl*
anticancer anticancéreux/anticancéreuse
anticoagulant anticoagulant *m*
anticoagulant anticoagulant,-e
antidiarrheic antidiarrhéique *m*
antidote antidote *m*
antiemetic antivomatif *m*
antifreeze antigel *m*
antifungal antifongique
antigène m antigène *m*
antigenic antigénique
antihistamine antihistaminique *m*
antihistaminic antihistaminique *m*
anti-inflammatory anti-inflammatoire
antineoplastic anticancéreux/anticancéreuse
antipyretic antipyrétique
anti-rabies vaccine vaccin *m* contre la rage
antiseptic antiseptique *m*
antiseptic compress compresse *f* désinfectante
antiseptic cream crème *m* antiseptique
antiseptic liquid liquide *m* antiseptique
antiseptic wipe lingette *f* antiseptique
antiserum antisérum *m*
antitetanus serum sérum *m* antitétanique
antitoxic antitoxique

anti-toxin antitoxine *f*
antitussive antitussif/antitussive
antiviral antiviral,-e
anuresis anurie *f*
anuria anurie *f*
anus anus *m*
anxiety anxiété *f*
aorta aorte *f*
aortic isthmus isthme *m* aortique
apathy apathie *f*
aplastic anaemia anémie *f* aplasique
aplastic anaemia anémie *f* aplastique
apoplexy, stroke apoplexie *f*
appetency appétence *f*
apple pomme *f*
apply, to appliquer
appointment rendez-vous *m*
appropriate approprié,-e
aqueous humour humeur *f* aqueuse
arachidonic acid acide *m* arachidonique
arch of the eyebrow arcade *f* sourcilière
arterial embolism embolie *f* artérielle
arterioscelerosis artériosclérose *f*
arteritis artérite *f*
artery artère *f*
arthritis arthrite *f*
arthrocentisis arthrocentèse *f*
Arthropoda Arthropodes *mpl*
articular cartilage cartilage *m* articulaire
artificial feeding allaitement *m* artificiel
artificial heart valve prothèse *f* valvaire
artificial heart valve valve *f* artificielle
artificial insemination insémination *f* artificielle
artificial respiration respiration *f* artificielle
ascarid ascaride *m*
asleep endormi,-e
aspergillosis aspergillose *f*
asphyxia asphyxie *f*
aspirin poisoning intoxication *f* d'aspirine
assessment bilan *m*
assisted ventilation respiration *f* assistée

astasia-abasia astasie-abasie *f*
asthenia asthénie *f*
asthenic asthénique
asthma asthme *m*
astringent astringent
at grass au pré
ataxia ataxie *f*
ataxic ataxique
atelectasis atélectasie *f*
atlas atlas *m*
atomiser/spray vapo *m*
atomiser/spray vaporisateur *m*
atopy atopie *f*
atrophy atrophie *f*
atrophy, to atrophier
attack crise *f*
auboise aubiose *m*
Aujeszky's disease maladie *f* d'Aujeszky
aural haematoma hématome *m* auriculaire
aural resection résection *f* auriculaire
auricle oreillette *f* (du cœur)
auricular scabies gale *f* auriculaire
autogenic autogène
autogenous autogène
autogenous vaccine vaccin *m* autogène
auto-immunity auto-immunité *f*
autolysis autolyse *f*
automatic waterer abreuvoir *m* automatique
autotoxin autotoxine *f*
average moyen/moyenne
avian flu grippe *f* aviare
aviary volière *f*
awn (barb) barbelure *f*
axillaries axillaires *fpl*
axillary artery artère *f* axillaire
azoospermatism azoospermatisme *m*
azoospermia azoospermie *f*
azoturia myglobinurie *f*

B

babesiosis babésiose *f*
baby rabbit lapereau *m*
baby rat raton *m*
bacillus bacille *m*
back dos *m*
back at the knee genoux *mpl* creux
back, to reculer
bacteria bactéries *fpl*
bacterial dermatosis dermatoses *fpl* bactériennes
bacterial infection infection *f* bactérienne
bacula os *m* pénien
bad breath halitose *f*,
bad breath mauvaise haleine *f*
balance aplomb *m*
balance équilibre *m*
balanitis babinebalanite *f*
balanoposthitis balano-posthite *f*
ball and socket joint joint à rotule *m*
bandage, to mettre un bandage
bar barre *f*
barbed wire fil *m* de fer barbelé
barium enema lavement *m* baryté
bastard wing aile *f* bâtarde
bath baignoire *f*
bath bain *m*
bath, to baigner
bath, to donner un bain
be afraid/frightened, to avoir peur
be cold, to avoir froid
be disturbed, to s'agiter
be hot, to avoir chaud
be in pain, to avoir mal
be in pain, to souffrir
be infected, to s'infecter
be restless, to s'agiter
be sick, to vomir
be trapped,to être coincé,-e
beak, bill bec *m*

bearing edge surface *f* portante
become cancerous se cancériser
become chapped, to se crevasser
become worse, to dégrader
bed lit *m*
bedsore eschare *f*
bee abeille *f*
bee sting piqûre *f* d'abeille
behave, to se comporter
behaviour comportement *m*
belly ventre *m*
benign bénin, bénigne
best age for reproduction âge *m* idéal de reproduction
beta-carotene béta-carotène *m*
better mieux, meilleur
BHS streptocoque *m* béta-hémolytiques
biceps brachial muscle muscle *m* biceps brachial
bicoloured bicoloré,-e
bile bile *f*
biliverdin biliverdine *f*
bill (money) facture *f*
biopsy biopsie *f*
bird flu grippe *f* aviare
birth canal filière *f* pelvienne
bit mors *m*
bitch chienne *f*;femelle *f*
bite morsure *f*
bite, to mordre
black patches in the coat taches *fpl* noires dans le pelage
blacksmith forgeron *m*
bladder vessie *f*
bladder infection infection *f* de la vessie
bleed, to saigner
bleeding saignement *f*
blepharitis blépharite *f*
blind aveugle
blindness cécité *f*
blinkers œillères *fpl*
bloat dilatation-torsion *f* de l'estomac
bloating ballonements *mpl*
block, to (pain) neutraliser

blockage blocage *m*
blockage occlusion *f*
blocked nose nez *m* bouché
blood sang *m*
blood check bilan *m* sanguin
blood clot caillot *m* sanguin
blood flow flux *m* sanguin
blood poisoning empoisonnement *m* du sang
blood pressure tension *f*
blood sample prise *f* de sang
blood sugar level sucre *m* dans le sang
blood test analyse *f* de sang
blood transfusion perfusion *f* sanguine
blood vessel vaisseau *m* sanguin
bloodshot injecté,-e de sang
bloody stools selles *fpl* sanguinolentes
body corps *m*
bone os *m*
bone deformity déformation *f* osseuse
bone growth développement *m* osseux
bone marrow moelle *f* osseuse
bone spavin eparvin *m* calleux
bony enlargement développement *m* osseux
booster injection piqûre de rappel
boredom ennui *m*
borreliosis borréliose *f*
bottom lip lèvre *f* inférieure
bowel intestins *mpl*
bowel movement selles *fpl*
box (plant) buis *m*
boxy feet pied *m* de pinçard
bracken fougère *f*
bradycardia bradycardie *f*
bradycardia bradyrythmie *f*
bradycardiac bradycardique
brain cerveau *m*
brain lesion lésion *f* cérébrale
break in a horse, to débourrer un chevel
break in, to débourrer
breaking in (a horse) débourrage *m*
breaking of the waters perte *f* des eaux

breaking of the waters rupture *f* de la poche des eaux
breast poitrail *m*
breastplate collier *m* de poitrine
breath haleine *f*
breathe, to respirer
breathing respiration *f*
breech presentation présentation *f* postérieure
breeder éleveur *m*
breeding élevage *m*
breeding plumage plumage *m* nuptial
bridle bride *f*
bridle a horse, to brider un cheval
brisket bréchet *m*
brochitis bronchite *f*
broken cassé,-e
bronchiolitis bronchiolite *f*
bronchopneumonia broncho-pneumonie *f*
bronchus bronche *f*
brood mare poulinière *f*
brooding, incubation couvaison *f*
brucellosis brucellose *f*
bruise contusion *f*
brush the teeth, to brosser les dents
brush, to brosser
brushing brossage *m*
brushing boots bottes *fpl* de canon
budgerigar perruche *f*
budgie perruche *f*
build gabarit *m*
bulging eyeballs yeux *mpl* globuleux
bulky stools selles *fpl* volumineuses
burn brûlure *f*
burn ointment pommade *f* contre les brûlures
burning brûlant,-e
burr épillet *m*
bursitis hygroma *m*
burst blood vessel vaisseau *m* éclaté
bushy touffu,-e
buttercup bouton *m* d'or
buttock fesse *f*
by mouth par voie *f* orale

41

C

cachexia cachexie *f*
"cactus" cloth chiffon *m* "cactus"
caecum caecum *m*
caesarean section césarienne *f*
cage cage *f*
cage size dimensions *fpl* de la cage
calcanean tuber tuberosité *f* du calcanéus
calcaneus calcanéum *m*
calcemia calcémie *f*
calcium calcium *m*
calf knees genoux *mpl* de *m*outon
calling en chaleur
callus callosité *f*
Campylobacter pylori Helicobacter pylori
cancer cancer *m*
cancerous cancéreux/cancéreuse
cancerous cells cellulles *fpl* cancérisées
candida candidose *f*
Candida albicans Candida albicans
canine canin,-e *adj*
canine distemper maladie *f* de Carré
canine herpes virus herpèsvirus *m* canin
canine kennel cough tracheobronchite *f* infectieuse
canine parvovirus infection parvovirose *f*
canine tooth canine *f*
cannabilism cannabalisme *m*
cannon bone canon *m*
cannon's circumference tour *m* du canon
canter petit gallop *m*
canter, to aller au petit gallop
capillary vaisseau *m* capillaire
capped elbow éponge *f*
capped hock capelet *m*
capsule gelule *f*

carbohydrates féculents *mpl*
carbon monoxide poisoning intoxication *f* par oxyde de carbone
carcinogenic cancérigène
carcinogenic cancérogène
carcinoma carcinome *m*
cardiac cardiaque
cardiac arrythmia arythmie *f* cardiaque
cardiac insufficiency insuffisance *f* cardiaque
cardiomyopathy cardiomyopathie *f*
cardio-vascular diseases maladies *fpl* cardio-vasculaires
cardiovascular system système *m* cardio-vasculaire
carditis cardite *f*
caress caresse *f*
carnivore carnivore *m*
carnivorous carnivore
carotid artery artère *f* carotide
carpal bones os *mpl* du carpe
carpus carpe *m*
carrying case caisse *f* de transport
cartilage cartilage *m*
castor oil huile *f* de ricin
castrated castré,-e
castration castration *f*
cat chat *m*; chatte *f*
cat litter, bedding (horses) litière *f*
cat mint herbe *f* aux chats
cat nip herbe *f* aux chats
cat scratch disease bartonellose
catabolism catabolisme *m*
cataract cataracte *f*
catarrh catarrhe *m*
catarrhal catarrhal,-e
catch, to attraper
catheter sonde *f*
catheterization cathétérisme *m*
catheterization sondage *m*
catheterize, to sonder
caudal caudal,-e
caudal tibial artery artère *f* tibiale caudale
caudal vertebrae vertèbres *fpl* caudales
cauterisation cautérisation *f*

43

cauterise, to cautériser
cautery cautère *m*
cavity cavité *f*
cell cellule *f*
cellulitis cellulite *f*
cement (tooth) cément *m* (dent)
central nervous system système *m* nerveux central
cereals céréales *fpl*
cereals graines *mpl*
cerebellum cervelet *m*
cerebral cérébral,-e
cerebral cortex cortex *m* cérébral
cerebral embolism embolie *f* cérébrale
cerebral vascular accident CVA accident *m* vasculaire cérébral AVC
cerebrospinal cérébro-spinal,-e
cerebro-spinal fluid liquide *m* céphalo-rachidien
cervical spondylitis spondylite *f* cervicale
cervical vertebrae vertébres *fpl* cervicales
cervix col *m* d'utérus
Cestoda Cestodes *mpl*
chafing frottant,-e contre
chalazion chalazion *m*
chap, to crevasser
chapped fendillé,-e
charcoal charbon *m* de bois
check, to vérifier
cheek ganache *f*
cheek joue *f*
cheek pouches bajoues *fpl*
cheilitis cheilite *f*
chemist pharmacien *m* pharmacienne *f*
chemist's shop pharmacie *f*
chemosis chémosis *m*
chest poitrail *m*
chestline poitrine *f* inférieure
chestnut châtaigne *f*
chew, to mordiller
chew, to ronger
cheyletiella infection cheyletiellose *f*
chiggers; harvest ticks aoûats *mpl*
chill refroidissement *m*

chin menton *m*
chin groove barbe *f*
chirp, to gazouiller
chlorine chlore *m*
choke, to s'étrangler
choking suffocation *f*
cholecystitis cholécystite *f*
choline choline *f*
chondrodysplasia chondrodysplasie *f*
chondrodysplasia chondrodystrophie *f*
chorea chorée *f*
choriomeningitis chorio-méningite *f*
choroid choroïde *f*
chromosome chromosome *m*
chromosomic aberration aberration *f* chromosomique
chronic chronique
chronic disease maladie *f* chronique
chronic enteritis entérite *f* chronique
chronic obstructive pulmonary disease (COPD) insuffisance *f* pulmonaire chronique
chronic rhinitis rhinite *f* chronique
chylothorax chylothorax
ciliary body corps *m* ciliaire
circulation circulation *f*
cirrhosis cirrhose *f*
claw griffe *f*
claw ongle *m*
clean propre
clean, to nettoyer
clear, to (nose, chest etc) dégager
cleft palate palais *m* fendu
climb, to grimper
cloaca cloaque *m*
clone clone *m*
clot caillot *m*
coagulant coagulant *m*
coagulation coagulation *f*
coat (of animal) pelage *m*
coat (of animal) robe *f*
cob cob *m*
coccidiosis coccidiose *f*

congenital deformity

cochlear cochléaire
cockatoo cacatoès *m*
coffin joint articulation *f* du pied
coitus coït *m*
cold froid,-e
cold (illness) rhume *m*
cold pack emplâtre *m*
cold to the legs froid *m* aux jambes
colibacillosis colibacillose *f*
colic colique *f*
colitis colite *f*
collapse collapsus *m*
collapsed trachea collapsus *m* tracheal
collarbone clavicule *f*
collie eye anomaly CEA anomalie *f* de l'œil du colley
colon côlon *m*
colostomy colostomie *f*
colostrum colostrum *m*
colprocele colprocèle *m*
colt poulain *m*
comatose comateux/comateuse
coming-in of milk montée *f* de lait
common calcanean tendon tendon *m* calcanéen commun
common digital extensor muscle muscle *m* extenseur dorsal du
    doigt
common digital flexor tendon tendon *m* du fléchisseur superficiel
common digital flexor tendon tendon *m* du perforé
communication communication *f*
complementary medicine médicine *f* douce
complications complications *fpl*
compress compresse *f*
concentrate (food) concentré *m*
concentrates concentrés *mpl*
conception conception *f*
concussion commotion *f*
concussion commotion *f* cérébrale
confusion confusion *f*
congenital congénital,-e
congenital cerebellar hypoplasis hypoplasie *f* cérébelleuse
    congenitale
congenital deformity difformité *f* congenitale

congenital dislocation of the patella luxation *f* congénitale de la
otule
congentital heart malformation malformation *f* cardiaque
congénitale
congestion congestion *f*
conjunctivitis conjonctivite *f*
constant constant,-e
constant habituel,-elle
constipated constipé,-e
constipation constipation *f*
consultation consultation *f*
consulting room cabinet *m*
contagion contagion *f*
contagious contagieux/contagieuse
contagious illness maladie *f* contagieuse
continually growing teeth dents *fpl* à croissance continue
contraceptive implant implant *m* contaceptif
contraceptive pill pilule *f* contraceptive
contraction contraction *f*
contraindication contre-indication *f*
control of the horse contrôle *m* du cheval
control, to contrôler
convulsion convulsion *f*
cool off refroidir
cooler couverture *f* de refroidissement
cooperative coopératif/coopérative
copper cuivre *m*
coprophagy coprophagie *f*
corn (on foot) cor *m*
cornea cornée *f*
corneal dystrophy dystrophie *f* cornéenne
corner (teeth) coin *m* (dent)
corner of mouth commissure *f* de la bouche
coronary body bourrelet *m* principal
coronary corium bourrelet *m* principal
coronary groove gouttière *f* cutigérale
coronary thrombosis infarctus *m*
coronary vein veine *f* coronaire
coronet couronne *f*
correct level niveau *m* approprié
corrosive corrosif/corrosive

corticosteroids corticostéroïdes *mpl*
corticotherapy corticothérapie *f*
cortisone cortisone *f*
coryza, cold in the head coryza *m*
cotton bud bâtonnet *m* de coton
cotton wool coton *m*
cotton wool ouate *f*
cover a mare, to saillir une jument
covert bars barres *fpl* alaires
cow hocks jarrets *mpl* clos
cow hocks jarrets *mpl* de vache
crack, to se crevasser
cramp crampe *f*
cranial tibial artery artére *f* tibiale crâniale
cream crème *m*
cremation incinération *f*
crepe bandage bande *f* Velpeau
crest of neck encolure *f*
crib biting tic *m* à l'appui
crib biting tic *m* aérophagique
crisis crise *f*
crop jabot *m*
cross-breeding croisement *m*
crossed croisé,-e
croup croupe *f*
crown sommet *m* de la tête
cruciate ligaments ligaments *mpl* croisés
crushing écrasement *m*
cryptosporidiosis cryptosporidiose *f*
curable guérissable
curb bit mors *m*
cure remède *m*
cure, to guérir
curry comb étrille *f*
curry, to étriller
curvature déviation *f*
Cushing's disease maladie *f* de Cushing
cut incision *f*
cut pad coussinet *m* déchiré
cut, to couper
cut, to inciser

cutaneous cutané,-e
cutting of the ears otectomie *f*
cutting teeth poussées *fpl* dentaires
cuttlefish bone os *m* de seiche
cyanosed mucus membranes muqueuses *fpl* cyanosées
cyanosis cyanose *f*
cyst kyste *m*
cysthostomes cysthominés *mpl*
cystotomy cystotomie *f*

D

daily care soins *mpl* quotidiens
damp humide
dampness humidité *f*
dancing mouse souris *f* danceuse
dandelion pissenlit *m*
dandruff pellicules *fpl*
dangling ears oreilles *fpl* tombantes
dead décédé,-e
dead mort,-e
deaf sourd,-e
deafness surdité *f*
decongestant décongestif *m*
decongestant décongestionnant *m*
decontamination décontamination *f*
deep digital flexor tendon tendon *m* du fléchisseur profond
deep digital flexor tendon tendon *m* du perforant
deep inguinal ring anneau *m* inguinal profond
deer cerf *m*; chevreuil *m*
defecate, to déféquer
defecation défécation *f*
defect tare *f*
deficiency carence *f*
degeneration, dégénération *f*
degenerative myelopathy myélopathie *f* dégénérative
deglutition déglutition *f*
dehydrate, to se déshydrater

diabetic

dehydrated déshydraté,-e
deltoid muscle muscle *m* deltoïde
demodecia démodecie *f*
demodetic mange demodecie *f*
demodex démodex *m*
dental calculus plaque *f* dentaire
dental plaque plaque *f* dentaire
dental problem maladie *f* péridontale
dental treatment traitement *m* dentaire
dentine dentine *f*
dentine ivoire *m* de la dent
depigmentation of the muzzle dépigmentation *f* du museau
depression abattement *m*
dermatitis dermatite *f*
dermatitis dermite *f*
dermatomycosis dermatomycose *f*
dermatophytes dermaophytes *mpl*
dermatophytosis dermatophytie *f*
dermatophytosis dermatophytose *f*
dermis derme *m*
dermoid cyst kyste *m* dermoïde
dermoid of the cornea dermoïde *m* cornéen
descaling détartrage *m*
descending colon côlon *m* descendant
destructive destructeur/destructrice
detached placenta décollement *m* du placenta
detached retina décollement *m* de la rétine
detect, to (disease etc) dépister
deteriorate, to se dégrader
deteriorating sight vue *f* abîmée
deterioration dégénérescence *f*
detoxification désintoxication *f*
detoxify, to désintoxiquer
develop, to évoluer
deviation déviation *f*
dewclaw ergot *m*
dewlap fanon *m*
diabetes diabète *m*
diabetes insipidus diabète *m* insipide
diabetes mellitus diabète sucré
diabetic diabétique

diagnose, to diagnostiquer
diagnosis diagnose *f*
diagnosis diagnostic *m*
diagnostic diagnostique
dialysis dialyse *f*
diaphragm diaphragme *m*
diarrhoea diarrhée *f*
diathermy diathermique *f*
diet régime *m*
dietary fibre fibres *m* alimentaires
difficult difficile
difficult pénible
difficulty in urinating difficultés *fpl* pour uriner
digest, to digérer
digestible digestible
digestion digestion *f*
digestive problems troubles *mpl* digestifs
digestive system appareil *m* digestif
digestive system système *m* digestif
digital cushion coussinet *m* plantaire
digital pad coussinet *m* digité
dilated cardiomyopathy cardiomyopathie *f* dilatée
dilation dilitation *f*
dilation of the left atrium cordis dilitation *f* de l'oreillette gauche
dilation of the right atrium cordis dilitation *f* de l'oreillette droite
diplegia diplégie *f*
dipylidium caninum dipylidium caninum *m*
dirofilariosis dirofilariose *f*
dirty sale
dirtying malpropreté *f*
discharge écoulements *mpl*
discharge pertes *fpl*
discharge from the vulva écoulement *m* vulvaire
disease maladie *f*
disinfect, to désinfecter
disinfectant désinfectant *m*
dislocate, to se déboiter
dislocate, to se disloquer
dislocated eyeball luxation *f* du globe oculaire
dislocation dislocation *f*
dislocation of the patella luxation *f* de la rotule

disobedience désobéissance *f*
disorder désordre *m*
displace, to déplacer
displacement déviation *f*
distal sesamoid petit sésamoïde *m*
distended gonflé,-e
distension gonflement *m*
distichiasis distichiasis *f*
distinguishing the sexes différenciation *f* des sexes
diuretic diurétique *m*
diurnal diurne
dizziness vertige *m*
dock coire *f*
dock of tail base *f* de la queue
docking of the tail caudectomie *f*
doctor docteur *m*
doctor médecin *m*
dog chien *m*; chienne *f*
domesticated apprivoisé,-e
donkey âne *m*
dorsal dorsal,-e
dorsal vertebra vertèbre *f* dorsale
dosage posologie *f*
drain, to drainer
drain, to vidanger
drainage tube, drain drain *m*
draughts courants *mpl* d'air
draw the pus, to aspirer le pus
dress, to (wound etc) panser
dressing pansement *m*
dribble, to baver
drink boisson
drink, to boire
drip feeding drip *m* feeding
drool, to baver
drop goutte *f*
dropper compte-gouttes *m*
dropping crottin *m*
dropping (a foal) mise-bas *f*
droppings (of bird) fiente *m*
drown, to se noyer

drowning noyade *f*
drug drogue *f*
dry cough toux *f* sèche
dry eyes sécheresse *f* des yeux
dry food croquettes *fpl*
dry keratoconjunctivitis kérato-conjonctivite *f* sèche
dry nose museau *m* sec
dry nose truffe *f* sèche
dry skin peau *f* désechée
dry, to sécher
dull coat robe *f* terne
dung crottin *m*
duodenitis duodénite *f*
duodenum duodénum *m*
dwarf rabbit lapin *m* nain
dyslipemia dyslipémie *f*
dyslipemia dyslipidémie *f*
dysphagia dysphagie *f*
dysplasia dysplasie *f*
dyspnea dyspnée *f*
dystocia dystocie *f*
dysuria dysurie *f*

E

ear oreille *f*
ear canker otite *f* externe
ear cleaning nettoyant *m* auriculaire
ear coverts parotiques *fpl*
ear coverts zone *f* auriculaire
ear drops gouttes *fpl* pour les oreilles
ear drum tympan *m*
ear flap pavillon *m*
ear mites acariens *mpl* auriculaires
ear mites otocariose *f*
earache mal *m* à l'oreille
early précoce
early diagnosis diagnostic *m* précoce
earwax bouchon *m* de cire
earwax cérumen *m*
easily assimilated assimilable
easily digested tolerance *f* digestive

easy facile
eating habits façon *m* de *m*anger
eating habits habitudes *fpl* alimentaires
echinococcosis échinococcose *f*
eclampsia éclampsie *f*
ectopic testicle ectopie *f* testiculaire
ectropion ectropion *m*
effectiveness efficacité *f*
efficacy efficacité *f*
effleurage effleurage *m*
egg œuf *m*
elbow coude *m*
elbow joint articulation *f* du coude
electric groomer pansage *m* électrique
electric shock décharge *f* électrique
electrocardiogram ECG électrocardiogramme *m* ECG
electrocardiograph ECG électrocardiographie *f* ECG
electrocution électrocution *f*
electroencephalogram EEG électroencéphalogramme *m* EEG
electroencephalogram EEG électroencéphalographie *f* EEG
electrolytes électrolytes *mpl*
electronic chip puce *f* électronique
eliminate, to éliminer
elimination élimination *f*
Elizabethan collar collerette *f*
elongated soft palate allongement *m* du voile du palais
emaciated amaigrissé,-e
emaciation amaigrissement *m*
emaciation emaciation *f*
embolism embolie *f*
embrocation embrocation *f*
embryo embryon *m*
embryonic embryonnaire
emergency urgence *f*
emergency treatment médecine *f* d'urgence
emetic emétique *m*
empty, to vidanger
encephalitis encéphalite *f*
encephalomyelitis encéphalomyélite *f*
encopresis encoprésie *f*
endemic endémique

endemic disease endémie *f*
endocarditis endocardite *f*
endocrine glands glandes *fpl* endocrines
endometritis endométrite *f*
endometrium endomètre *m*
endoscope endoscope *m*
endoscopy endoscopie *f*
endurance résistance *f*
enema lavement *m*
engorge, to engorger
engorgement engorgement *m*
enriched with enrichi,-e de
enteritis entérite *f*
enterotomy entérotomie *f*
enterotoxemia entérotoxémie *f*
enterovirus entérovirus *m*
entrocolitis entérocolite *f*
entropion entropion *m*
enuresis enurèse *f*
enuresis enurésie *f*
enzootic enzootique
enzyme enzyme *m*
epidemic épidémie *f*
epidermis épiderme *m*
epididymitis epididymite *f*
epiglottis épiglotte *f*
epilepsy épilepsie *f*
epiphora epiphora *m*
epispadias epispadias *m*
epistaxis epistaxis *f*
epithelial dystrophy dystrophie *f* épithéliale
Epsom salts sels *mpl* d'Epsom
epulis épulis *m*
equestrian équestre
equine équin,-e; chevalin,-ine; équidé
equine glanders morve *f*
equine infectious anemia anémie *f* infectieuse équine
equine influenza grippe *f* équine
equine oxyuris oxyuridés *mpl*
equine strongyloidosis strongylose *f* équine
equine veterinarian vétérinaire *m* de chevaux

external

equipment équipement *m*
equitation équitation *f*
eradicate éradiquer
eradication éradication *f*
erysipelas érisipèle *m*
erysipelas érysipèle *m*
erythema érythème *m*
erythrocyte globule *m* rouge
erythrocyte hématie *f*
erythrocyte érythocyte *m*
erythrocyte sedimentation rate vitesse *f* de sédimentation globulaire
erythrocyte sedimentation rate vitesse *f* de sédimentation sanguine
essential essentiel/essentielle
essential epilepsy épilepsie *f* esentielle
essential fatty acids acides *mpl* gras essentiels
ethmoid(al) labyrinth labyrinthe *m* ethmoïdal
ethmoid(al) labyrinth labyrinthe *m* olfactif
ethylene glycol éthylène *m* glycol
Eustachian tube trompe *f* d'Eustache
euthanasia euthanasie *f*
eutocia eutocie *m*
evolve, to évoluer
ewe neck encolure *f* de cerf
examination examen *m* medical
examine, to faire un examen
excess dose surdosage *m*
excitability nervosité *f*
excite to exciter
excressance excroissance *f*
excreta excreta *m*
excrete, to excréter
excretion excrétion *f*
exercise exercice *m*
exercise bandage bande *f* de travail
exhaustion abattement *m*
exhaustion épuisement *m*
expectorant expectorant,-e
external externe
external bleeding hémorragie *f* externe
external ear oreille *f* externe
external iliac artery artère *f* iliaque externe

external thoracic artery artère *f* thoracique externe
extract, to (tooth etc) arracher
extract, to (tooth etc) extraire
extraction extraction *f*
extrasystole extrasystole *f*
eye drops collyre *m*
eye injuries blessures *fpl* aux yeux
eye lotion collyre *m*
eye ring cercle *m* orbital
eye; eyes œil *m*; yeux *mpl*
eyebrow sourcil *m*
eyedrops gouttes *fpl* pour les yeux
eyelash cil *m*
eyelid paupière *f*
eye-stripe bandeau *m* sur l'œil

F

face visage *m*
facial paralysis paralysie *f* faciale
facial eczema eczéma *m* faciel
faeces fèces *fpl*
faint, to s'évanouir
fall chute *f*
fall, to tomber
Fallopian tube trompe *f* de fallope
false pregnancy grossesse *f* nerveuse
Faradism faradisation *f*
farrier maréchal-ferrant *m*
fast jeûne *m*
fast, to jeûner
fatal mortel/mortelle
fatal illness maladie *f* mortelle
fatigue fatigue *f*
fats matières *fpl* grasses
fatty cyst kyste *m* graisseux
fatty tumour tumeur *f* graisseuse
faulty heart rhythm rythme *m* anormal de cœur
feacal analysis analyse *f* de selles
fear peur *m*

feather plume *f*
feather lice poux *mpl* de plumes
feather loss chute *f* de plumes
feather-plucking picage *m*
fecal incontinence incontinence *f* fécale
fecaloma fecalome *m*
feed alimentation *f*
feed, to (by the mother) téter
feeding pattern régime *m* alimentaire
feeding tube sonde *f* d'alimentation
feline félin,-ine
feline calicivirus calicivirose *f*
feline chlamydial infection chlamydiose *f*
feline dysautonomia dysautonomie *f* féline
feline endocrine alopecia alopécie *f* endocrinienne féline
feline eosinophilic syndrome syndrome *m* éosinophilique félin
feline hemobartonellosis hémobartonellose *f* féline
feline immunodeficiency virus immunodéficience *f* féline
feline infectious anaemia anémie *f* infectieuse féline
feline infectious enteritis typhus *m*
feline infectious peritonitis (PIF) péritonite *f* infectieuse féline
feline leukaemia virus leucose *f* féline
feline panleucopaenia panleucopénie *f*
feline pneumanitis pneumonite *f* féline
feline respiratory disease complex rhino-trachéite *f* infectieuse féline
feline rodent ulcer complexe granulome *m* eosinophilique félin
feline scabies gale *f* de la tête
feline urological syndrome (FUS) sablose *f*
female femelle *f*
female rabbit lapine *f*
female rat ratte *f*
femoral fémoral,-e
femur fémur *m*
ferment, to fermenter
ferret furet *m*
fertile fécond,-e
fertilisation fécondation *f*
fertilised fécondé,-e
fertility fertilité *f*
fetlock boulet *m*

fetlock boots protèges-boulets *mpl*
fetlock joint articulation *f* du boulet
fever fièvre
feverish fiévreux/ fiévreuse
fibre fibre *m*
fibrocartilage fibrocartilage *m*
fibroid fibrome *m*
fibroma fibrome *m*
fibrosarcoma fibrosarcome *m*
fibula fibula *m*
field of view champ *m* visuel
file dossier *m*
filly pouliche *f*
fire incendie *f*
fireworks feux *mpl* d'artifice
first-aid premiers soins *mpl*
fish poisson
fissure fissure *f*
fistula fistule *f*
fit crise *f* d'épilepsie
fit en pleine forme
flank flanc *m*
flat-sided plat dans ses arceaux
flea collar collier *m* anti-puces
flea powder poudre *f* anti-pouces
flea spray vaporisateur *m* anti-puces
fleas puces *fpl*
fleece toison *f*
flews babines *fpl*
flexion flexion *f*
flexion incurvation *f*
fly mouche *f*
fly repellent produit *m* anti-mouches
fly, to voler
foal poulain *m*
foal, to pouliner
foam écume *f*
foetal death mort *f* fœtale
foetal sac sac *m* anmiotique
foetus fœtus *m*
folic acid acide *m* folique

folliculitis folliculite *f*
food allergy allergie *f* alimentaire
food bowl écuelle *f*
food bowl gamelle *f*
food container mangeoire *f*
food poisoning intoxication *f* alimentaire
food supplement complément *m* alimentaire
foot pied *m*
foot and mouth disease fièvre *f* aphteuse
fore limb membre *m* antérieur
forearm avant-bras *m*
forecannon canon *m* antérieur
forechest poitrine *f* antérieure
forehand avant-main *f*
forehead front *m*
foreign body corps *m* étranger
forelock toupet *m*
forepaw patte *f* antérieure
form fiche *f*
founder fourbure *f*
foxglove digitale *f*
fracture fracture *f*
fractured fracturé,-e
fragile fragile
frequent vomiting vomissements *mpl* répétés
frog (on hoof) fourchette *f*
frontal bone os *m* frontal
frontal sinus sinus *m* frontal
frostbite gelure *f*
fruit fruit *m*
full of wax bouché,-e de cire
functional fonctionnel/ fonctionnelle
functioning fonctionnement *m*
fungal infection infection *f* fongique
fur fourrure *f*
fur ball boule *f* de poil
furuncle furoncle *m*
furonculosis furonculose *f*
furry ears oreilles *fpl* poilues

G

galactorrhea galactorhée *f*
gall bladder vésicule *f* biliaire
gall stone calcul *m* biliaire
gallop galop *m*
Gamgee tissue Gamgee *m*
gamma globulin gamma-globuline *f*
ganglion ganglion *m*
gangrene gangrène *f*
gaping béant,-e
garrot garrot *m*
gaskin jambe *f*
gastric gastrique
gastric ulcer ulcère *m* de l'estomac
gastritis gastrite *f*
gastroenteritis gastro-entérite *f*
geld, to castrer
gelding hongre *m*
gene gène *m*
general anaesthetic anasthésie *f* générale
general purpose polyvalent,-e
generalised mange démodécie *f* généralisée
genetic génétique
genital discharge perte *f* génitale
genital hypoplasia hypoplasie *f* génitale
genital infantilism infantilisme *m* genital
gerbil gerbille *f*
gerbil mérione *m* de *m*ongolie
germ carrier porteur *m* de germes
gestation gestation *f*
get slimmer, to s'amincir
giardia giardia *m*
giardiosis giardiose *m*
gingivitis gingivite *f*
girth sangle *f*
gizzard gésier *m*
gland glande *f*

glasspaper papier *m* de verre
glaucoma glaucome *m*
globulin globuline *f*
glomérulonephritis glomérulonéphrite *f*
glossitis glossite *f*
glucose glucose *m*
glycerine glycérine *f*
glycerine glycérol *m*
glycosuria glycosurie *f*
goitre goitre *m*
gonad gonade *f*
good health bonne santé *f*
gout goutte *f*
goutte à goutte f drip
granulation tissue bourgeonnement *m* d'une plaie
granulocyte granulocyte *m*
granuloma granulome *m*
grass herbe *f*
grass sickness mal *m* de l'herbe
graze, to brouter
graze, to paître
grazing patûrage
greater coverts grandes couvertures *fpl*
greenery verdure *f*
greenish discharge pertes *fpl* verdâtres
greenstick fracture fracture *f* incomplète
grind the teeth, to grincer les dents
grit gravillons *mpl*
groin aine *f*
groom palefrenier *m*
groom valet d'écurie *m*
groom, to panser
grooming toilette *f*
grooming (dog) toilettage *m*
growth croissance *f*
grunting grognement *m*
guard dog chien *m* de garde
guarding its territory protection *f* territoriale
guinea pig cochon *m* d'inde
gum gencive *f*
gun dog chien *m* de chasse

gynaecomastia gynécomastie *f*

H

hack hack *m*
hack to se promener à cheval
haemarthrosis hémarthrose *f*
haematemesis hématémèse *f*
haematology hématologie *f*
haematoma hématoma *m*
haematuria hématurie *f*
haemoglobin hémoglobine *f*
haemoglobinuria hémaglobinurie *f*
haemolysis hémolyse *f*
haemoperitoneum hémoperitoine *m*
haemophilia hémophilie *f*
haemoptysis hémoptysie *f*
haemorrhage hémorragie *f*
haemostasis hémostase *f*
hair poil *m*
hair follicle follicule *m* pileux
halt to faire halt
halter licol *m*
hamster hamster *m*
hand rear, to nourrir à la main
handle, to manipuler
hard dur,-e
hard hat casque *m* protecteur
hard skin couche *f* cornée
Harderian gland glande *f* de Harder
harelip bec-de lièvre *m*
harness harnais *m*
have a high temperature, to avoir de la fièvre
have a relapse, to avoir/faire une rechute
have a relapse, to rechuter

hay foin *m*
hay bale balle *f* de foin
hay fever rhume *m* des foins
hay rack râtelier *m* à fourrage
haylage herbe *m* en sac plastique
haynet filet *m* à foin
hazelnut noisette *f*
head tête *f*
head presentation présentation *f* antérieure
headache mal *m* de tête
healing guérison *f*
healing (of wound etc) cicatrisation *f*
health check bilan *m* de santé
health record carnet *m* de santé
hearing audition *f*
hearing problems troubles *mpl* de l'audition
heart cœur *m*
heart beat pulsation *f*
heart disease maladie *f* du cœur
heart failure arrêt *m* du cœur
heart murmur bruits *mpl* cardiaques
heart rate rythme *m* cardiaque
heat stroke coup *m* de chaleur
heavy lourd,-e
heavy salivation salivation *f* abondante
hedge haie *f*
heel talon *m*
hemlock ciguë *f*
heparin héparine *f*
hepatic failure insuffisance *f* hépatique
hepatitis hépatite *f*
herbivorous herbivore
herd harde *f*
hereditary illness maladie *f* héréditaire
hereditary trait affection *f* héréditaire
heredity hérédité *f*
hermaphrodism hermaphrodisme *m*
hernia hernie *f*
herpes herpès *m*
herring-gutted ventre *m* de levrette
hibernate, to hiberner

hibernation hibernation *f*
highly digestible hautement digestible
highly strung nerveux/nerveuse
hign temperature forte température *f*
hind limb membre *m* postérieur
hind-cannon canon *m* postérieur
hip bone os *m* iliaque
hip dysplasia dysplasie *f* de la hanche
hip joint articulation *f* de la hanche
histiocytoma histiocytome *m*
hob mâle *m* furet
hock (joint) jarret *m*
hock boots protèges-jarrets *mpl*
hock, point of pointe *f* du jarret
hogged mane crinière *f* rase
hollow ensellement *m*
hoof sabot *m*
hoof horn corne *f*
hoof pick cure-pied *m*
hookworm ankylostome *f*
hookworm disease ankylostomose *f*
horizontal external ear canal conduit *m* auditif externe horizontal
hormonal disturbance déreglement *m* hormonal
hormonal fluctuation fluctuation *f* hormonale
hormone hormone *m*
hormone treatment traitement *m* hormonal
Horner's syndrome syndrome *m* d'Horner
hornet frelon *m*
horny sole sole *f* cornée
horse cheval *m*
horse bot gastrophile *m*
horse dentist dentiste *m* équin
horse nuts granules *mpl* à cheveaux
horsetails prèles *fpl*
hot chaud,-e
household bleach eau *f* de Javel
house-trained propre
how to take (drugs etc) mode *f* et voie *f* d'administration
howl, to hurler
humerus humérus *m*
hunter chasseur *m*

hunting dog chien *m* de chasse
hurt oneself, to se blesser
hurt oneself, to se faire mal
hydrocele hydrocèle *f*
hydrogen peroxide eau *f* oxygénée
hydronephrosis hydronéphrose *f*
hydrotherapy hydrothérapie *f*
hygiene hygiène *f*
hygiene soins *mpl* d'hygiène
hypercalcemia hypercalcémie *f*
hyperlipaemia hyperlipémie *f*
hyperlipaemia hyperlipidémie *f*
hyperplasia hyperplasie *f*
hypertension hypertension *f* artérielle
hyperthermia hyperthermie *f*
hyperthyroidism hyperthyroïdie *f*
hyperthyroidism hyperthyroïdisme *m*
hypertrophic osteodystrophy osteodystrophie *f* hypertrophique
hypertrophy hypertrophie *f*
hypervitaminosis hypervitaminose *f*
hypogcalcemia hypocalcémie *f*
hypoglycemia hypoglycémie *f*
hypokalaemic polymyopathy polymyopathie *f* hypokaliémique
hypokalemia hypokaliémie *f*
hypoplasia hypoplasie *f*
hypospadias hypospadias *m*
hypothermia hypothermie *f*
hypothyroidism hypothyroïdie *f*
hypoxia hypoxie *f*
hysterectomy hystérectomie *f*

I

iatrogenic iatrogène
iatrogenic iatrogénique
ichtyosis ichtyose *f*
ideal weight poids *m* idéal

identification papers papiers *fpl* d'identification
identity ring bague *f* d'identification
idiopathic idiopathique
ileitus iléite *f* proliférative
ileus ileus *m*
iliac iliaque
iliac artery artère *f* iliaque
iliac thrombosis thrombose *f* iliaque
ilium os *m* ilium
ill health maladie *f*
ill-health mauvaise santé *f*
illness maladie *f*
imbalance of hormones déséquilibres *mpl* hormonaux
immobilise, to immobiliser
immune system système *m* immunitaire
immunisation immunisation *f*
immunisation against immunisation *f* contre
immunity immunité *f*
impacted pouches bajoues *fpl* collées
impetigo gourme *f*
impetigo impétigo *m*
in captivity en captivité
in season en chaleur
inappetence inappétence *f*
inborn defect tare *f* héréditaire
inbreeding couplement *m* consanguin
incisor dent *f* incisive
incisor incisive *f*
incontinence incontinence *f*
incoordination incoordination *f*
increase, to augmenter
increasing temperature augmentation *f* de la température
increasing thirst augmentation *f* de la soif
incubation period période *f* d'incubation
indication indication *f*
indigestion dyspesie *f*
indigestion indigestion *f*
induce labour, to déclencher l'accouchement
induced labour accouchement *m* déclenché
infected infecté,-e
infected bite morsure *f* infectée

67

insufficiency

infection infection *f*
infection of the ventral sebaceous gland infection *f* de la glande sébacée ventrale
infectious infectieux/ infectieuse
infectious canine hepatitis hépatite *f* contagieuse
infectious disease maladie *f* transmissible
infectious illness maladie *f* infectieuse
infertile stérile
infertility infertilité *f*
infest, to infester
infestation infestation *f*
infested infesté,-e
inflamed enflammé,-e
inflammation inflammation *f*
inflammation of the uterus inflammation *f* de l'uterus
inflammatory inflammatoire
in-foal pleine
information renseignements *mpl*
infrared lamp lampe *f* infrarouge
infrared light rayons *mpl* infrarouge
ingredients composition *f*
inguinal glands glandes *fpl* inguinales
inhale inhaler
inhaler inhalateur *m*
inhibitor inhibiteur *m*
inhibitory inhibiteur/ inhibitrice
inject (to) injecter
injection injection *f*
injure oneself, to se blesser
injure, to blesser
injured blessé,-e
injury blessure *f*
inner ear oreille *f* interne
inquisitive curieux/curieuse
insect bite piqûre *f*
insect repellant insectifuge *m*
insecticide antiparasitaire *m*
insecticide insecticide *m*
insert a catheter into mettre une sonde à
insomnia insomnie *f*
insufficiency insuffisance *f*

insulin insuline *f*
insurance assurance *f*
intelligent intelligent,-e
intensive care réanimation *f*
interdigital cyst kyste *m* interdigité
interdigital pyoderma pyodermite *f* interdigitée
interferon interféron
interior internal,-e
intermission intermission *f*
intermittant intermittent,-e
internal internal,-e
internal interne
internal bleeding hémorragie *f* interne
internal iliac artery artère *f* iliaque interne
internal injuries lésions *fpl* internes
internal thoracic artery artère *f* thoracique interne
intertrigo intertrigo *m*
intervene, to intervenir
intervention intervention *f*
intestinal blockage occlusion *f* intestinale
intestinal disorders désordres *mpl* intestinaux
intestinal flora flore *f* intestinale
intestinal parasites parasites *mpl* intestinaux
intestinal perforation perforation *f* intestinale
intestine intestin *m*
intolerance of intolérance *f* à
intradermic injection injection *f* intradermique
intramuscular intramusculaire
intramuscular injection injection *f* intramusculaire
intranasal intranasal,-e
intraocular intraoculaire
intraocular pressure pression *f* intraoculaire
intraocular pressure tension *f* intraoculaire
intraocular pressure tension *f* oculaire
intrauterine intra-uterin,-e
intravenous intraveineux/intraveineuse
intravenous injection injection *f* intraveineuse
intubation intubation *f*
invagination invagination *f*
invasive invasif/invasive
inversion déviation *f*

69

juvenile

involution involution *f*
iodine iode *m*
iridocyclitis iridocyclite *f*
iris iris *m*
iritis iritis *f*
iron fer *m*
irradiated irradié,-e
irradiation irradiation *f*
irreversible damage dégâts *mpl* irréversibles
irrigate, to irriguer
irrigation irrigation
irrigator irrigateur *m*
irritant irritant *m*
irritant irritant,-e
irritated gums irritation *f* des gencives
irritation irritation *f*
isolate, to isoler
isolated isolé,-e
isolation isolation *f*
isthmus of the thyroid isthme *m* thyroïdien
isthmus of the uterus isthme *m* de l'utérus
itch démangéaison *f*
itch, to démanger

J

jaundice ictère *m*
jaundice jaunisse *f*
jaw mâchoire *f*
jill femelle *f* furet
joint articulation *f*
joint joint *m*
jowl bajoue *f*
jugular groove sillon *m* jugulaire
jugular vein veine *f* jugulaire
jump, to sauter
juvenile petit *m*

K

kalemia kaliémie *f*
kaolin kaolin *m*
Kaposi's sarcoma sarcome *m* de Kaposi
kennel chenil *m*
kennel cough toux *f* de chenil
keratin kératine *f*
keratinisation kératinisation *f*
keratitis kératite *f*
keratoconjunctivitis kérato-conjonctivite *f*
keratosis kératose *f*
kerion kérion *m*
Key-Gaskell syndrome syndrome *m* de Key-Gaskell
kick, to botter
kidney rein *m*
kidney failure insuffisance *f* rénale
kidney stones calcul *m* rénal
kit (ferret) bébé *m* furet
kitten chaton *m*
knackers yard équarrissage *m*
knead, to piétiner
kneading piétinement *m*
knee genou *m*
knot nœud *m*

L

labour travail *m*
laburnum cytise *f*

lazy digestion

lacerate, to déchirer
laceration déchirure *f*
lachrymal ducts conduits *mpl* lachrymaux
lachrymal gland glande *f* lacrymale
lachrymatory ducts conduits *mpl* lachrymaux
lack of carence *f* de
lack of carence *f* en
lack of manque *m* de
lack of appetite manque *f* d'appétit
lack of exercise manque *m* d'exercice
lack of exercise manque *m* d'exercice
lack of hygiene manque *m* d'hygiène
lacrimal bone os *m* lacrimal
lactation lactation *f*
lameness boiterie *f*
laminar corium chorion *m* de la paroi
laminitis laminite *f*
lance bistouri *m*
lance lancette *f*
lance, to ouvrir
lance, to percer
laparostomy laparostomie *f*
laparotomy laparotomie *f*
large grand,-e
large breed dogs chiens *mpl* de grand race
large metatarsal bone os *m* métatarsien principal
large red worm grand ver *m* rouge
large strongyles grands strongles *mpl*
large tooth-comb démêloir *m*
larva larve *f*
laryingitis laryngite *f*
laryngospasm laryngospasme *m*
larynx larynx *m*
lateral crown stripe bandeau *m* de la tête
lateral digital extensor muscle muscle *m* extenseur latéral du doigt
lateral ligament ligament *m* latéral
laurel laurier *m*
laxative laxatif *m*
laxity laxité *f*
lay an egg, to pondre
lazy digestion digestion *f* paresseuse

lead laisse *f*
lead plomb *m*
lead poisoning saturnisme *m*
lead poisoning colic coliques *fpl* de plomb
left auricle oreillette *f* gauche
left bronchus bronche *f* gauche
left pulmonary artery artère *f* pulmonaire gauche
left side côté *m* gauche
left ventral colon côlon *m* ventral gauche
left ventricle ventricule *m* gauche
left-overs restes *mpl*
leg jambe *f* (horse)
leg patte *f* (animal)
leg bandage bande *f* de travail
leishmaniasis leishmaniose *f*
length longeur *m*
length of pregnancy durée *f* de gestation
lens cristallin *m*
lens luxation luxation *f* de cristallin
leptospirosis leptospirose *f*
lesion lésion *f*
lesser coverts petites couvertures *fpl*
lethergy léthargie *f*
leucism leucisme *m*
leucocyte leucocyte *m*
leucocytosis leucocytose *f*
leucorrhea leucorrhée *f*
leucosis leucose *f*
lice poux *mpl*
lick, to lécher
life expectancy longévité *f*
ligament ligament *m*
ligature ligature *f*
light leger/legère
light massage effleurage *m*
limp claudication *f*
limp, to boîter
linoleic acid acide *m* linoléïque
lip lèvre *f*
lipoma lipome *m*
liquid paraffin huile *f* de paraffine

73

lump

lithiasis lithiase *f*
litter (of kittens etc) portée *f*
litter (for cat) litière *f*
litter tray bac *m* à litière
liver foie *f*
liver disease maladie *f* du foie
local anaesthetic anasthésie *f* locale
localised mange démodécie *f* localisée
locked/tied mating nœud *m* sexual
locomotor ataxia ataxie *f* locomotrice
locum remplaçant *m* remplaçante *f*
loin reins *mpl*
long claws griffes *fpl* longues
long pastern bone os *m* du paturon
longevity longévité *f*
long-haired à poil long
look after, to soigner
loosebox box *m*
lore lorums *mpl*
lose consciousness, to perdre connaissance
lose its appetite, to pedre l'appetit
lose one's appetite, to perdre l'appétit *m*
lose weight, to s'amaigrir
loss of appetite manque *f* d'appétit
loss of appetite perte *f* d'appétit
loss of balance perte *f* d'équilibre
loss of blood perte *f* de sang
loss of body fat dégénérescence *f* graisseuse
loss of consciousness perte *f* de connaissance
loss of hair/fur dépilation *f*
loss of hearing perte *f* d'auditon
loss of weight amaigrissement *m*
lower inférieur,-e
lower eyelid paupière *f* inférieure
lower incisor incisive *f* inférieure
lower jaw mâchoire *f* inférieure
lower lobe (lung) lobe *m* inférieur
lower the temperature, to baisser la température
lower thigh jambe *f*
lumbar vertebrae vertèbres *fpl* caudales lombaires
lump bosse *f*

lump grosseur *f*
lung poumon *m*
lupus lupus *m*
lymph lymphe *f*
lymph glands ganglions *m* lymphatiques
lymph node ganglion *m* lymphatique
lymphangitis lymphangite *f*
lymphatic system système *m* lymphatique
lymphocyte lymphocyte *m*
lymphoedema lymphoedème *m*
lymphosarcoma lymphosarcome *m*
lymphosarcomatosis lymphosarcomatose *f*
lysosomal disease maladie *f* lysosomale

M

macula degeneration dégénérescence *f* maculaire
magnesium magnésium *m*
make sore, to blesser
male mâle *m*
malformation of the tail déformation *f* de la queue
malignancy malignité *f*
malignant malin, maligne
mallassezia mallassezia *m*
malnutrition sous-alimentation *f*
malocclusion malocclusion *f* dentaire
mammary glands glandes *fpl* mammaires
mammary hypertrophy hypertrophie *f* mammaire
mammary tumour tumeur *m* mammaire
mandible mandibule *f*
mane crinière *f*
mane pulling comb peigne *m* à tirer la crinière
manganese manganèse *m*
mange gale *f*
manger auge *f*
manipulation manipulation *f*

membrane

mantle manteau *m*
manure fumier *m*
marasmus marasme *m*
mare jument *f*
mare in foal jument *f* gestante
mark, to marquer
marking of territory marquages *m* de territoire
masseter muscle muscle *m* masseter
mastitis mammite *f*
mastitis mastite *f*
mastosis mastose *f*
mate, to se coupler
mating accouplement *m*
mating saillie *f*
mating season rut *m*
matted fur poils *mpl* collés
mauled mutilé/e
maxilla maxillaire *m*
maxillary maxillaire
maximum maximum
meadow hay foin *m* du pré
meadow saffron colchique *m*
meat viande *f*
medial head of the deep digital flexor muscle muscle *m* fléchisseur médial du doigt
medial ligament ligament *m* médial
median coverts couvertures *fpl* moyennes
median crown stripe bande *f* cranienne
mediastinitis médiastinite *f*
mediastinum médiastin *m*
medication medication *f*
medicine médecine *f*
medicine (treatment) medicament *f*
medium moyen/ moyenne
medullary aplasia aplasie *f* médullaire
megacolon mégacôlon *m*
megaoesophagus mégalooesophage *m*
megaoesophagus mégaoesophage *m*
melanin mélanine *f*
melanoma mélanome *m*
membrane membrane *f*

Ménière's disease maladie *f* de Ménière
meninges méninges *fpl*
meningitis méningite *f*
meningocele méningocèle *f*
metabolism métabolisme *m*
metacarpal métacarpien/ienne
metacarpal pad coussinet *m* métacarpien
metacarpal pad coussinet *m* palmaire
metacarpus métacarpe *m*
metal mane comb peigne *m* en métal
metaplasis métaplasie *f*
metastasis métastase *f*
metatarsal métatarsien/métatarsienne
metatarsal bones os *mpl* du métatarse
metatarsal pad coussinet *m* métatarsien
metatarsal pad coussinet *m* plantaire
metatarsus métatarse *m*
method méthode *f*
metrorrhagia métrorragie *f*
metrorrhea métrorrhée *f*
mew, to miauler
miaow, to miauler
microchip puce *f* électronique
micropore tape sparadrap *m* microporeux
micturition miction *f*
middle ear oreille *f* moyenne
middle lobe (lung) lobe *m* moyen
middle phalanx phalange *f* intermédiaire
miliary dermatitis dermatite *f* miliare
milk lait *m*
milk tooth dent *f* de lait
millet millet *m*
minimum minimum
miosis myosis *m*
miscarriage fausse-couche *f*
mismating mésalliance *f*
mites acares *mpl*
mitral endocardiosis endocardiose *f* mitrale
mixomatosis mixomatose *f*
modification modification *f*
moist food aliment *m* humide

molar molaire *f*
mongrel bâtard *m*
monitor, to surveiller
monitoring surveillance *f*
monkshood aconit *m*
monocyte monocyte *m*
monocytosis monocytose *f*
monorchidia monorchidie *f*
moonblindness uvéite *f* récidivante
morphine morphine *f*
mosquito repellent produit *m* antimoustique
motor system appareil *m* locomoteur
moult, to muer
moulting mue *f*
mouse souris *f*
moustachial stripe moustache *f*
mouth bouche *f*
mouth gueule *f*
mouth to mouth resuscitation bouche-à-bouche *m*
mouth ulcer aphte *m*
muck out, to nettoyer
mucocele mucocèle *f*
mucus mucus *m*
mud fever infection *f* cutanée bactérienne
mule mule *m*
muscle muscle *m*
muscular rupture rupture *f* musculaire
mustang mustang *m*
mute muet/muette
muzzle or nose (of horse) chanfrein *m*
muzzle museau *m*
muzzle (strap or wire) muselière *f*
myasthenia myasthénie *f*
myasthenia gravis myasthénie *f*
mycetoma mycétome *m*
mycosis fungoides mycosis *f* fongoïde *f*
mycosis, fungal infection mycose *f*
mycotoxicosis mycotoxicose *f*
mycotoxin mycotoxine *f*
mydriasis mydriase *f*
myelitis myélite *f*

myeloma myélome *m*
myelopathy myélopathie *f*
myiasis myiase *f*
myocarditis myocardite *f*
myocardium myocarde *m*
myopathy myopathie *f*
myopia myopie *f*
myopic myopique
myositis myosite *f*
myotonia myotonie *f*

N

nail ongle *m*
nail bed matrice *f* unguéale
nail clipping coupe *f* des ongles
nail-clipper coup-ongle *m*
nametag médaille *f*
narcolepsy narcolepsie *f*
narcosis narcose *f*
narrow at the chest serré,-e de poitrail
nasal cavity cavité *f* nasale
nasal discharge écoulement *m* nasal
nasolacrimal duct conduit *m* naso-lacrymal
nasolacrimal duct deformity difformité *f* de la voie nasolacrymale
national stud farm haras *m* national
natremia natrémie *f*
natural defences défenses *fpl* naturelles
nausea nausée *f*
navicular bone os *m* navicular
navicular syndrome maladie *f* naviculaire
necessary nécessaire
neck cou *m*
neck encolure *f*
neck nuque *f*
necropsy autopsie *f*
necrosis nécrose *f*

necrosis of the cornea nécrose *f* de la cornée
neigh, to hennir
neighing hennissement *m*
neonatal néonatal,-e
neoplasia néoplasie *f*
neoplastic néoplasique
nephritis néphrite *f*
nephrosis néphrose *f*
nerve nerf *m*
nervous afflictions affections *fpl* nerveuses
nervous disposition tempérament *m* nerveux
nest nid *m*
nestbox nichoir *m*
nestling oisillon *m*
neurodermatosis neurodermatose *f*
neurological neurologique
neutered châtré,-e
neutralise, to neutraliser
niacin niacine *f*
nibble, to grignoter
nibble, to mordiller
nictating membrane membrane *f* nictatante
night blindness hemeralopie *f*
nightshade belladone *f*
nipple mamelon *m*
nocturnal nocturne
nodule nodule *m*
noisy bruyant,-e
non-inflammatory arthritis arthrose *f*
normal wear and tear usure *f* normale
nose chanfrein *m*
nose nez *m*
nose truffe *f*
noseband muserolle *f*
nosebleed saignement *m* de nez
nosedrops gouttes *fpl* pour le nez
nostril narine *f*
nostril naseau *m*
numbness engoudissement *m*
nutriment nutriment *m*
nutrition nutritition *f*

nutritional needs besoins *mpl* nutritionnels
nutritious nourrissant/e
nutritious nutritif,nutritive
nyctalopia nyctalopie *f*
nymphomania nyphomanie *f*
nystagmus nystagmus *m*

O

obedience obéissance *f*
obesity obésité *f*
observation observation *f*
observe, to observer
obstruct, to engorger
obstructed tear ducts obstruction *f* des voies lacrymales
obstruction engorgement *m*
obstruction of the intestines occlusion *f* intestinale
occasional occasionel,-e
occiput occiput *m*
occlude, to occlure
occlusion occlusion *f*
oedema œdème *m*
oesophagitis œsophagite *f*
oesophagus œsophage *m*
oestrogen œstrogène *m*
oestrus œstrus *m*
oestrus control réglementation *f* d'œstrus
offensive-smelling stools selles *fpl* malodorantes
oil huile *f*
ointment pommade *f*
oleander laurier *m* rose
olecranon olécrâne *m*
olfactory olfactif/olfactive
oliguria oligurie *f*
omnivorous omnivore
omphalitis ompalite *f*
on an empty stomach jeun; à jeun
on heat en chaleur

on the sole of the foot plantaire
onychitis onyxis *m*
oophorectomy ovariectomie *f*
oophorohysterectomy ovario-hystérectomie *f*
opaque opaque
operation opération *f*
ophthalmia ophtalmie *f*
ophthalmoscope ophtalmoscope *m*
ophthalmoscopy ophtalmoscopie *f*
optic nerve nerf *m* optique
optic neuritis névrite *f* optique
oral oral,-e
oral cavity cavité *f* buccale
oral hygiene hygiène *f* buccale
orchitis orchite *f*
organ organe *m*
orthopedics orthopédie *f*
oslerosis oslérose *f*
osteitis ostéite *f*
osteo-arthritis of the hip arthrose *f* de la hanche
osteochondritis ostéochondrite *f*
osteochondrosis ostéochondrose *f*
osteofibrosis ostéofibrose *f*
osteolysis ostéolyse *f*
osteomyelitis ostéomyélite *f*
osteopathy ostéopathie *f*
osteoporosis ostéoporose *f*
osteosarcoma osteosarcome *m*
othematoma othématome *m*
otoscopy otoscopie *f*
ototoxicity ototoxicité *f*
outer primary coverts couvertures *fpl* marginales
outgrowth excroissance *f*
ovarian cyst kyste *m* ovarien
ovariectomy ovariectomie *f*
ovariohysterectomy ovario-hystérectomie *f*
ovary ovaire *m*
over at the knee genoux *mpl* brassicourts
over dose surdose *f*
overactive adrenal glands hyperfonctionnement *m* des surrénales
overdosage surdosage *m*

overeating suralimentation *f*
overheat, to échauffer
overpopulation surpopulation *f*
overreach s'atteindre en talon
overreach boots cloches *fpl*
overtraining surentraînement
overweight surpoids
ovulate ovuler
ovulation ovulation *f*
ovum ovule *m*
owner propriétaire *m*
oxygen oxygène *m*

P

pacemaker pacemaker *m*
pacemaker stimulateur *m* artificiel
pacemaker stimulateur *m* cardiaque
pachymeningitis méningite *f* externe
pachymeningitis pachyméningite *f* ossifante
pad coussinet *m*
pad, carpal/stopper coussinet *m* carpien
pad, dew coussinet *m* de l'ergot
paddock sheet chemise *f* de paddock
pain douleur *f*
painkiller calmant *m* analgésique
painkilling antalgique
pale gums gencives *fpl* pâles
palpate, to palper
panarteritis panartérite *f*
panarthritis panarthrite *f*
pancreas pancréas *m*
pancreatitis pancréatite *f*
panniculitis panniculites *fpl*

83

panophtalmia panophtalmie *f*
pansteatitis panstéatite *f*
pant, to haleter
panting halètement *m*
papillomatosis papillomatose *f*
parakeet perruche *f* ondulée
paralysed paralysé,-e
paralysis paralysie *f*
paraphimosis paraphimosis *m*
paraplegia paraplégie *f*
parasite parasite *m*
parasitic otitis otite *f* parasitaire
parasitosis parasitose *f*
parathyroid gland glande *f* parathyroïde
paresis parésie *f*
paronychia paronychie *f*
parrot perroquet *m*
parturition parturition *f*
pastern métacarpe *m*
pastern paturon *m*
pasteurellosis pasteurellose *f*
patella rotule *f*
patella ligament ligament *m* rotulien
pathological laboratory (path lab) laboratoire *m* pathalogique
paw patte *f*
pay, to payer
peanuts cacahuètes *fpl*
peat moss tourbe *f*
pedal bone os *m* du pied
pedal bone rotation rotation *f* de l'os du pied
pedalosteitis ostéite *f* de la troisième phalange
pedigree certificat *m* d'ascendence
pedigree pedigree *m*
pelvic cavity cavité *f* pelvienne
pelvis bassin *m*
pemphigus pemphigus *m*
penis pénis *m*
penis bone os *m* pénien
peptic ulcer ulcère *m* duodénal
perch perchoir *m*
perch, to se percher

perforation perforation *f*
pericardal cavity cavité *f* péricardique
pericardium péricarde *m*
peridontitis parodontite *f*
peridontium paradonte *m*
peridontium paradontium *m*
peridontosis paradontose *f*
perinatal périnatal,-e
perineum périnée *m*
periodontal disease parodontite *f*
perionyxis périonyxis *m*
periople périople *m*
perioplic ring bourrelet *m* périoplique
periostitis périostite *f*
periostium périoste *m*
periostosis périostose *f*
peristaltis péristaltisme *m*
peritoneal cavity cavité *f* péritoneale
peritoneum péritoine *m*
peritonitis péritonite *f*
perk up, to se réquinquer
perleche perlèche *f*
permanent tooth dent *f* permanente
permit licence *f*
pernicious anaemia anémie *f* pernicieuse
pernicious anaemia maladie *f* de Biermer
persistant wound démangeasion *f* persistante
perspiration/sweat perspiration *f*
perspiration/sweat sueur *f*
perspiration/sweat transpiration *f*
pessary ovule *m*
pessary pessaire *m*
pet animal *m* de compagnie
pet cemetery cimetière *m* animalier
pet insurance assurance *m* animaux de compagnie
Pet's Passport Programme *m* de Voyage des Animaux de Compagnie (PVAC)
phalanx prima première phalange *f*
phalanx secunda deuxième phalange *f*
phalanx tertia troisième phalange *f*
phantom pregnancy grossesse *f* nerveuse

85

pharmacy pharmacie *f*
pharyngitis pharyngite *f*
pharynx pharynx *m*
pheromone phéromone *f*
phimosis phimosis *m*
phlebitis phlébite *f*
phlegmon phlegmon *m*
phobia phobie *f*
phosphorus phosphore *m*
photophobia photophobie *f*
phtirioses phtiriose *f*
physiotherapy kinésithérapie *f*
pica pica *m*
pick out a foot, to curer un pied
pigeon toes pieds *mpl* cagneux
pigment pigment *m*
pill comprimé *m*
pill pilule *f*
pin worm oxyure *m*
pinna pavillon *m*
pinning (bone etc) brochage *m*
piroplasmosis piroplasmose *f*
pituitary gland glande *f* pituitaire
placenta placenta *m*
plait, braid tresse *f*
plait, braid, to tresser
plaited forelock toupet *m* tressé
plaited mane crinière *f* tressée
plaited tail queue *f* tressée
plasma plasma *m*
plaster (for break, fracture) plâtre
plastic wedge cale *f* en plastique
platelet thrombocyte *m*
platelets plaquettes *fpl*
pleural cavity cavité *f* pleurale
pleural effusion epanchement *m* pleural
plumage plumage *m*
plumbism saturnisme *m*
plump enrobé,-e
plumpness embonpoint *m*
pneumonia pneumonie *f*

86

pneumothorax pneumothorax *m*
point of buttock pointe *f* de la fesse
point of hip pointe *f* de la hanche
point of shoulder pointe *f* de l'épaule
poison poison *m*
poison (snake) venin *m*
poison, to empoisonner
poisoned bait appât *m* empoisoné
poisoning empoisonnement *m*
poisonous nocif/nocive
poisonous toxique
poisonous plant plante *f* toxique
poisonous spider araignée *f* venimeuse
poll nuque *f*
pollakiuria pollakisurie *f*
pollakiuria pollakiurie *f*
polo pony poney *m* de polo
polyarthritis polyarthrite *f*
polydactyly polydactylie *f*
polydactyly polydactylisme *m*
polydipsia polydipsie *f*
polymyositis polymyosite *f*
polyp polype *m*
polyphagy polyphagie *f*
polyuria polyurie *f*
polyuria-polydipsia polyuro-polydipsie *f*
pommel pommeau *m*
pony poney *m*
pooper scooper Pooper Scooper *m*
poor hearing audition *f* abîmée
poor socialisation manque *m* de socialisation
posology posologie *f*
posterior chamber of the eye chambre *f* postérieure de l'œil
posthitis posthite *f*
post-mortem autopsie *f*
postnatal postnatal
potassium potassium *m*
potomania potomanie *f*
poultice cataplasme *m*
powder poudre *f*
poxvirus poxvirus *m*

protein

preen, to lisser
pregnancy gestation *f*
pregnant gravide
pregnant pleine
premature ageing vieillissement *m* prématuré
premolar prémolaire *f*
preparation for the birth préparation *f* de la couche
prescription ordonnance *f*
prevent, to prévenir
preventative measures mesures *fpl* préventives
priapism priapisme *m*
primaries (feathers) rémiges *fpl* primaires
primary coverts couvertures *fpl* primaires
primary osteoarthritis arthrose *f* primaire
primary vaccination primo-vaccination *f*
privet troène *m*
procidentia procidence *f*
procidentia of the third eyelid procidence *f* de la troisième paupière
proctitis proctite *f*
profound cervical artery artère *f* cervicale profonde
progeny testing épreuve *f* sur/de la descendance
progesterone progestérone *f*
prognathic prognathe
prognosis prognostic *m*
prognosis pronostic *m*
progressive évolutif/évolutive
progressive pernicious anaemia anémie *f* pernicieuse progressive
prolapse prolapsus *m*
prolapse of the eyeball prolapsus *m* du globe oculaire
prolapse of the rectum prolapsus *m* du rectum
pro-oestrus pro-œstrus *m*
prophylaxis prophylaxie *f*
proprietary food aliment *m* industriel
prostate prostate *m*
prostate cancer cancer *m* de la prostate
prostate gland enlargement adénome *m* de la prostate
prostatectomy prostatectomie *f*
prostatism prostatisme *m*
prostatitis prostatite *f*
prosternum pointe *f* du sternum
protein protéine *f*

proteinuria protéinurie *f*
prothesis prothèse *f*
proven stallion/sire étalon *m* qui a fait ses preuves
provide water, to abreuver
proximal phalanx phalange *f* proximale
proximal sesamoid grand sésamoïde *m*
pruriginous dermatosis dermatose *f* prurigineuse
pruritis prurit *m*
pseudogestation pseudogestation *f*
pseudotuberculosis pseudotuberculose *f*
psittacosis psittacose *f*
psychodermatoses psychodermatoses *fpl*
psychotropic psychotrope *m*
ptosis ptôse *f*
ptyalism ptyalisme *m*
puberty puberté *f*
pubic bone os *m* pubis
puerperal tetany tétanie *f* puerpérale
pull out, to arracher
pull, to tirer
pulled muscle claquage *m* musculaire
pulmonary pulmonaire
pulmonary artery artère *f* pulmonaire
pulmonary disease maladie *f* pulmonaire
pulmonary emphysema emphysème *m* pulmonaire
pulmonary lesion lesion *f* pulmonaire
pulmonary vein veine *f* pulmonaire
pulpitis pulpite *f*
pulse pouls *m*
puncture ponction *f*
puncture wound clou *m* de rue
puncture, to ponctionner
punctured percé,-e
pupil pupille *f*
puppy chiot *m*
pure alcohol alcool *m* absolu
pure breed de race
purgative purgatif *m*
purgative purgation *f*
purgative purge *f*
purpura purpura *m*

89

rash

purr, to ronronner
purulent purulent,-e
pus pus *m*
put a dressing on, to mettre un pansement sur
put down, to euthanasier
put on weight, to grossir
putting on muscle mise *f* en muscle
pyelonephritis pyélonéphrite *f*
pyloric sphincter sphincter *m* pylorique
pylorus pylore *m*
pyometra pyomètre *m*
pyorrhea pyorrhée *f*
pyrexia pyrexie *f*
pyuria pyurie *f*

Q

quarantine quarantaine *f*
quartering quartering *m*
quartering quartier *m*
queen chatte *f*
quittor javart *m* cartilagineux

R

rabbit lapin *m*
rabbit haemorraghic disease maladie *f* hemorragique virale
rabid enragé,-e
rabies rage *f*
radius radius *m*
ragwort jacobée *f*
rain scald échaudure *f*
rapid breathing respiration *f* accélérée
rare disease maladie *f* rare
rash éruption *f*

rat rat *m*
reaction réaction *f*
readjust, to réadapter
ready-made food aliments *mpl* tout prêts
rear pastern métatarse *m*
rear up, to cabrer
rear, to se cabrer
reception accueil *m*
recover récupérer
recovery guérison *f*
rectal ampulla ampoule *f* rectale
rectal examination toucher *m* rectal
rectal prolapse prolapsus *m* rectal
rectal temperature témperature *f* rectale
rectal thermometer thermomètre *m* rectal
rectal wall paroi *f* rectale
rectitis rectite *f*
rectum rectum *m*
recuperate récupérer
recur, to récidiver
recurrence récidive *f*
recurring récidivant,-e
red blood cells globules *mpl* rouge
reduced activity activité *f* réduite
reduced calorie food alimentation *f* light
reduced mobility mobilité *f* réduite
regain consciousness reprendre connaissance
regular brushing brossage *m* regulier
regurgitate régurgiter
regurgitation régurgitation *f*
rehabilitate rééduquer
rein guide *f*
re-infection réinfection *f*
relapse rechute *f*
relax relâcher
relaxation détente *f*
relieve congestion, to décongestionner
remove the droppings, to enlever les crottins
remove, to enlever
renal rénal,-e
renal colic colique *f* néphrétique

roll

renal diabetes diabète *m* rénal
resection résection *f*
respiration respiration *f*
respiratory allergy allergie *f* respiratoire
respiratory failure arrêt *m* respiratoire
respiratory rate fréquence *f* respiratoire
respiratory strongyles strongyles *fpl* respiratoires
respiratory system/tract appareil *m* respiratoire
respiratory system/tract système *m* respiratoire
rest repos *m*
rest, to reposer
resuscitation réanimation *f*
retention rétention *f*
retention of eggs rétention *f* d'œufs
retention of urine rétention *f* d'urine
retina rétine *f*
retinal atrophy atrophie *f* rétinienne
retriever chien *m* rapporteur
rhabdomyolysis rhabdomyolyse *f*
rheumatoid arthritis polyarthrite *f* rheumatoïde
rhinitis rhinite *f*
rhinopharyngitis rhinopharyngite *f*
rhododendron rhododendron *m*
rib côte *f*
ribcage cage *f* thoracique
rickets rachitisme *m*
rider cavalier *m*
right auricle oreillette *f* droite
right balance juste balance *m*
right bronchus bronche *f* droite
right pulmonary artery artère *f* pulmonaire droite
right side côté *m* droite
right ventral colon côlon *m* ventral droit
right ventricle ventricule *m* droit
rigor mortis rigidité *f* cadavérique
ringworm teigne *f*
rinse, to rincer
roach back dos *m* de mulet
road traffic accident accident *m* de la circulation
rodent rongeur *m*
roll, to se rouler

roller; surcingle surfaix *m*
roof of the mouth voûte *f* du palais
roof of the mouth voûte *f* palantine
rope burn prise *f* de longe
roughage fourrage *m*
rough-haired à poil *m* frisé
rounded rebondi,-e
roundworm ascaride *m*
roundworm toxocara
Rubarth's disease maladie *f* de Rubarth
rubber matting tapis *m* caoutchouc
rubber/latex gloves gants *mpl* latex
ruffled ébouriffé,-e
rug couverture *m*
rump croupe *f*
rump croupion *m*
run a temperature, to avoir de la fièvre
run, to (of eyes etc) couler
runny eyes écoulement *m* des yeux
rupture rupture *f*
ruptured rompu,-e

S

sacral vertebrae vertébres *fpl* sacrées
sacrum sacrum *m*
saddle selle *f*
saddle sore plaie *f* de selle
safety harnass harnais *m* de sécurité
saliva salive *f*
salivary cyst kyste *m* salivaire
salivary glands glandes *fpl* salivaires
salmonella salmonelle *f*
salmonellosis salmonellose *f*
salpingitis salpingite *f*
salt lick pierre *f* à lècher
sample prélèvement *m*
sand sable *m*

sandcrack seime *f*
sandpaper papier *m* de verre
sarcoidosis sarcoïdose *f*
saturnism saturnisme *m*
satyriasis satyriasis *m*
scab croûte *f*
scabies gale *f*
scalded ébouillanté,-e
scaling entartrement *m*
scan échographie *f*
scapula omoplate *f*
scapulars scapulaires *fpl*
scar cicatrice *f*
scent gland glande *f* anale
Scheuermann's disease maladie *f* de Scheuermann
sciatica sciatique *f*
scissors ciseaux *mpl*
sclera sclérotique *f*
sclerotomy sclérotomie *f*
scoot to se traîner l'arrière-train
scratch griffure *f*
scratching post griffoir *m*; griffure *f*
screening dépistage *m*
scrotum scrotum *m*
scurf peau *f* morte
sebaceous cyst kyste *m* sébacé
sebaceous cyst loupe *f*
sebaceous gland glande *f* sébacée
seborrhea séborrhée *f*
sebum sébum *m*
secondaries (feathers) rémiges *fpl* secondaires
secondary arthritis arthrose *f* secondaire
sedation sédation *f*
sedative sédatif *m*
seed hay foin *m* artificiel
seedy toe fourmilière *f* en pince
selenium sélenium *m*
self-adhesive bandage bandage *m* adhésif
self-sufficient autonome
semen semence *f*
semen sperme *m*

senility sénilité *f*
sense sens *m*
sense of smell odorat *m*
sensitive sensible
sensitive laminae chair *f* feuilletée
sensitive sole sole *f* sensible
sensitive stomach estomac *m* fragile
sepsis sepsie *f*
septic septique
septic arthritis arthrite *f* septique
septicaemia septicémie *f*
serology serologie *f*
Sertoli cell tumeur sertolinome *m*
serum sérum *m*
serving ration *f*
set on of tail base *f* de la queue
seton séton *m*
sexing sexage *m*
sexual maturity maturité *f* sexuelle
shadow on the lung voile *m* au poumon
shake its head, to secouer la tête
shake the ears, to secouer les oreilles
shake, to secouer
shallow breathing respiration *f* superficielle
shampoo shampooing *m*
sharp tranchant,-e
sharpen its claws, to aiguiser ses griffes
shave, to raser
shaved rasé,-e
sheath fourreau *m*
sheep dog chien *m* de berger
shelter abri *m*
shinbone tibia *m*
Shirmer's test test *m* de Shirmer
shiver frisson *m*
shiver with (shock etc), to grelotter de
shiver, to frissonner
shock choc *m*
shoe, to ferrer; (**shod** ferré,-e)
shoe (horse) fer *m*
shoeing ferrage *m*

shoes with rolled toes fers *mpl* à pince laminée
short pastern bone os *m* de la couronne
short-haired à poil court
shoulder épaule *f*
shoulder blade omoplate *f*
shoulder joint articulation *f* de l'épaule
shoulder joint pointe *f* du sternum
shredded paper papier *m* déchiqueté
shunt shunt *m*
sialitis sialite *f*
sialogenous sialogène
sialorrhea sialorrhée *f*
sickle hocks jarrets *mpl* coudés
sickness maladie *f*
side effects effets *mpl* non souhaités et gênants
side effects effets *mpl* secondaires
sidebone forme *f* cartiligineuse
sight problems troubles *mpl* de la vue
signs of ageing signes *mpl* de vieillissement
signs/indications of ear problems signes *mpl* auriculaires
signs/indications of eye problems signes *mpl* oculaires
signs indications of genital problems signes *mpl* génitaux
signs/indications of nervousness signes *mpl* nerveux
signs/indications of respiratory problems signes *mpl* respiratoires
signs/indications of urinary problems signes *mpl* urinaires
sing, to chanter
sinking affaissement *m*
sinusitis sinusite *f*
size taille *f*
skeletal frame ossature *m*
skeleton squelette
skin peau *f*
skin allergy allergie *f* cutanée
skin disease maladie *f* de peau
skittish nerveux/nerveuse
skull crâne *m*
slab-sided efflanqué
sleep through the night, to faire ses nuits
sleeping pill somnifère *m*
slim, to amaigrir
slipped disc hernie *f* locale

sloping shoulder épaule *f* inclinée
small petit,-e
small dogs chiens *mpl* de petite taille
small intestine intestin *m* grêle
small redworms petits strongyles *mpl*
small strongyles petits strongles *mpl*
smooth-haired à poil *m* lisse
snaffle mors *m* brisé
snaffle bit bride *f* à filet
snake bite (poisonous) morsure *f* de serpent (venimeux)
snake bite serum sérum *m* antivenimeux
sneeze éternuement *m*
sneeze, to éternuer
sneezing éternuements *mpl*
sniff, to renifler
snore, to ronfler
snoring ronflement *m*
snort, to s'ébrouer
soap savon *m*
sociable sociable
sodium sodium *m*
soft stools selles *fpl* molles
soiling malpropreté *f*
solar dermatitis dermatite *f* solaire
sole sole *f*
sole of the foot plante *f* de pied
solitary solitaire
sound (chest etc), to ausculter
spasm spasme *m*
spavins éparvins *mpl*
spay, to castrer
spay, to enlever les ovaries
spayed castré,-e
special precautions mises *fpl* en gardes spéciales
species espèce *f*
specimen prélèvement *m*
specimen (urine) échantillion *m*
speculum spéculum *m*
speed vitesse *f*
sperm sperme *m*
sperm analysis spermogramme *m*

97

sperm bank banque *f* de sperme
spike crampon *m*
spinabifida spina-bifida *m*
spinal cord cordon *m* médullaire
spinal cord colonne vertébrale *f*
spine colonne vertébrale *f*
splay-footed pieds *mpl* panards
spleen rate *f*
splenectomy splénectomie *f*
splenomegaly spléneomégalie *f*
splinter écharde *f*
splints (on a horse) suros *mpl*
spondylolisthesis spondylolisthésis *m*
spondylopathy spondylopathie *f*
sponge éponge *f*
sporadic sporadique
sprain entorse *f*
sprain, to se fouler
spray, to marquer
squamous cell carcinoma carcinome *m* squameux
squeal, to couiner
squint, to loucher
stable écurie *f*
stable bandage bande *f* de repos
stable equipment équipement *m* d'écurie
stale urine *f* (horse, cattle)
stale, to uriner
stall (horse) stalle *f*
stallion étalon *m*
stamina vigueur *f*
staphylococcus staphylocoque *m*
steatitis stéatite *f*
stenosis rétrécissement *m*
stenosis sténose *f*
step pas *m*
sterile compress tricostéril *m*
sterilizer sterilisateur *m*
sterilizing solution solution *f* de stérilisation
sternocephalicus muscle muscle *m* sterno-céphalique
sternum sternum *m*
sticking plaster pansement *m* adhésif

sticking plaster sparadrap *m*
stiffness raideur *f*
stifle grasset *m*
stifle joint articulation *f* du genou
stifle joint creux *m* du jarret
stillborn mort-né,-e
stimulate, to exciter
sting dard *m*
sting piqûre *f*
stinging nettle ortie *f*
stirrup étrier *m*
stitch suture *f*
stitch, to suturer
stomach estomac *m*
stomach ventre *m*
stomach pump pompe *f* stomachale
stomach tube sonde *f* gastrique
stomach wall paroi *f* intestinale
stomatitis stomatite *f*
stone pierre *f*
stones calculs *mpl*
stools selles *fpl*
stop stop *f*; cassure *f* du nez
strabismus strabisme *m*
strain a muscle, to se froisser un muscle
strained/pulled muscle élongation *f*
strangles gourme *f*
strangulated hernia hernie *f* étranglée
straw paille *f*
streptococci streptocoques *mpl*
stress stress *m*
stride foulée *f*
stroke attaque *f* cérébrale
stroke, to caresser
strongyloidosis vulgaris strongylose *f* vulgaris
stud farm haras *m*
stud horse reproducteur *m*
stud tail queue *f* grasse
stunted growth retard *m* de croissance
subacute subaigu/subaiguë
subclinical subclinique

sweat

subcutaneous sous-cutané,-e
subcutaneous injection injection *f* sous-cutanée
subcutaneous swellings gonflements *mpl* sous-cutanés
submission soumission *f*
submissive soumis,-e
suckle, to téter
sudden brutal,-e
suffer, to souffrir
suffocation étouffement *m*
suffocation suffocation *f*
sugar beet betterave *f* à sucre
suitable food for aliments *mpl* adaptés à
sulphonamides sulfamides *mpl*
sulphonamides sulfamidés *mpl*
summer coat robe *f* d'été
sun burn coup *m* de soleil
sunflower seeds graines *fpl* de tournesol
sunstroke insolation *f*
superficial superficiel,-e
superficial cervical artery artère *f* cervicale superficielle
superficial digital flexor muscle muscle *m* fléchisseur superficial du doigt
superficial gluteal muscle muscle *m* fessier superficial
superficial inguinal ring anneau *m* inguinal superficiel
supperating suppurant,-e
suppling assouplissement *m*
suppository suppositoire *m*
suppurative suppuratif/suppurative
suppurative suppuré,-e
supraorbital fossa salière *f*
surgery (place) cabinet *m*
surgery, operation chirurgie *f*
surgical spirit alcool *m* à 90
suspensory ligament ligament *m* suspenseur du boulet
suture suture *f*
swab tampon *m*
swallow, to avaler
sway back dos *m* fortement ensellé
sweat gland glande *f* sudoripare
sweat scraper couteau *m* de chaleur
sweat, to suer

sweet itch habronémose *f* cutanée
swell, to gonfler
swelling enflure *f*
swelling gonflement *m*
swollen balloné,-e
swollen gonflé,-e
symblepharon symblépharon *m*
symptom symptôme *f*
symptomatic symptomatique
syncope syncope *f*
syndrome syndrome *m*
synovial fluid liquide *m* synovial
synovial fluid synovie *f*
syringe seringue *f*
syringomyelia syringomyélie *f*

T

tachnypnoea tachypnée *f*
tachycardia tachyardie *f*
tack sellerie *f*
tail queue *f*
tail (rectrices) rectrices *fpl* externes
take out, to faire l'ablation de
take the bit in the teeth, to prendre le mors aux dents
take the temperature, to prendre la température
take to, to; to carry transporter
talon ongle *m*
tame apprivoisé,-e
tame,to apprivoiser
tapeworm ténia *m*
tarsal tarsien/tarsienne
tarsus tarse *m*
tartar tartre *m*
taste goût *m*
tattoo tatouage *m*

tattoo, to tatouer
tattooing tatouage *m*
taurine taurine *f*
tear déchirure *f*
tear duct conduit *m* lacrymal
tear, to (muscle etc) se déchirer
tear,to déchirer
teat mamelle *f*
teethe, to faire ses dents
temperament tempérament *m*
temperature température *f*
tendinitis tendinite *f*
tendon tendon *m*
tendon boots guêtres *fpl* de tendon
tendon bow claquage *m* de tendon
tenesmus ténesme *m*
teniasis téniasis *m*
tenosynovitis chauffage *m* de tendon
tenosynovitis téno-synovite *f*
teratogenic teratogène
terrarium terrarium *m*
test épreuve *f*, test *m*
test, to éprouver; tester
testicle testicule *m*
testosterone testostérone *f*
tetanus tétanos *m*
tetany tétanie *f*
tetracycline tétracycline *f*
thalamus thalamus *m*
thermometer thermomètre *m*
thiamin thiamine *f*
thiamin deficiency carence *f* de thiamine
thick fourni,-e
thick coat toison *f*
thigh cuisse *f*
thigh, lower jambe *m*
thigh, upper fémur
thighbone fémur *m*
thin the mane, to éclaircir la crinière
thin the tail, to éclaircir la queue
third eyelid troisième paupière *f*

thoracic aorta aorte *f* thoracique
thoracic cavity cavité *f* thoracique
thoracic vertebrae vertèbres *fpl* thoraciques
thorax thorax *m*
thorn épine *f*
thoroughbred de race
throat gorge *f*
throatlash gosier *m*
throatlash sous-gorge *f*
thrombosis thrombose *f*
thrombus thrombus *m*
throw the rider, to désarçonner le cavalier
thrush échauffement *f* de la fourchette
thrush muguet *m*
thymus thymus *m*
thyroid thyroïde *f*
tibia tibia *m*
tick tique *f*
tick remover crochet *m* à tiques
tied in below the knee poignets *mpl* étranglés derrière
time temps *m*
timid,frightened peureux/peureuse
tincture teinture *f*
tissue tissu *m*
titbits friandises *fpl*
toe pince *f*
toilet training apprentissage *m* de la propreté
tolerance tolérance *f*
tomcat matou *m*
tongue langue *f*
tonic tonique *m*
tonsillitis amygdalite *f*
tonsillitis angine *f*
too rich a diet alimentation *f* trop riche
tooth dent *f*
tooth decay carie *f*
tooth extraction avulsion *f* dentaire
tooth float blade lime *f* à dents
top coat poil *m* de couverture
top lip lèvre *f* supérieure
topical topique *f*

triscupiditis

torn déchiré,-e
torsion torsion *f*
torso torse *m*
toxaemia toxémie *f*
toxaemia in pregnancy toxemie *f* de gestation
toxicoderma toxicodermie *f*
toxicoderma toxidermie *f*
toxin toxine *f*
toxocara canis ascaris *m* du chien
toxocara cati ascaris *m* du chat
toxoplasma gondii toxoplasma gondii *mpl*
toxoplasmosis toxoplasmose *f*
toy dogs chiens *mpl* d'appartement
trachea trachée *f*
tracheitis trachéite *f*
tracheotomy trachéotomie *f*
train, to entraîner
training entraînement *m*
tranquillizer tranquillisant *m*
transmit, to se transmettre
transport, to transporter
trauma trauma *m*
traumatic depression enfoncement *m*
travel sickness mal *m* des transports
travelling boots guêtres *fpl* de voyage
travelling box boîte *f* de voyage
treat, to traiter
treatment traitement *m*
treats friandises *fpl*
tremor tremblement *m*
trichiasis trichiasis *m*
trichinosis trichinose *f*
trichobezoards trichobezoards *mpl*
trichonemes trichonèmes *mpl*
trim (hoof), to parer le sabot
trim the claws, to tailler les griffes
trimmed mane crinière *f* toilettée
trimming of the hoof parage *m* de la corne
tripe tripes *fpl*
triscupid valve valvule *f* triscupide
triscupiditis triscupidite *f*

trombiculosis trombiculose *f*
trot, to trotter
tuberculosis tuberculose *f*
tumour tumeur *f*
tweezers pincette *f*
twin jumeau *m* ; jumelle *f*
twins jumeaux *mpl* /jumelles *fpl*
typanism typanisme *m*
Tyzzer's disease maladie *f* de Tyzzer

U

ulcer ulcère *m*
ulcerate, to ulcérer
ulcerated ulcéré,-e
ulcerated cornea ulcère *m* de la cornée
ulcerated paws ulcération *f* des pattes
ulcerated wound plaie *f* ulcerée
ulceration ulcération *f*
ulna cubitus *m*
umbilical ombiliqué,-e
umbilical cord cordon *m* ombilical
umbilical hernia hernie *f* ombilicale
umbilicus ombilic *m*
unbalanced diet alimentation *f* déséquilibrée
unblock, to (intestine etc) libérer
uncinariasis ankylostamiase *f*
unconscious sans connaisance
under coat sous-poil *m*
underactive adrenal glands hypofonctionnement *m* des surrénales
underlying sous-jacent,-e
undertail coverts sous-caudales *fpl*
underweight maigre
uneven ondulant,-e
unnecessary pas nécessaire

unperforated tear ducts imperforation *f* des voies lacrymales
unpredictable imprévisible
unregistered sans papiers
unruly horse cheval *m* difficile
unsaddle, to desseller
unshod déférré,-e
unshoe, to déferrer
unusual inhabituel/inhabituelle
upper supérieur,-e
upper arm bras *m* supérieur
upper eyelid paupière *f* supérieure
upper incisor incisive *f* supérieure
upper jaw mâchoire *f* supérieure
upper lobe (lung) lobe *m* supérieur
upper thigh fémur *m*
uppertail coverts sus-caudales *fpl*
uraemia urémie *f*
urea urée *f*
ureter uretère *m*
ureteral ectopia éctopie *f* uréterale
urethral catheter sonde *f* urétale
uric acid acide *m* urique
urinary incontinence incontinence *f* urinaire
urinary tract voies *fpl* urinaires
urinate, to uriner
urine urine *f*
urine analysis analyse *f* d'urine
urolithiasis urolithiase
uropygial gland glande *f* uropygienne
urticaria urticaire *f*
use usage *m*
uterine inertia inertie *f* utérine
uterus utérus *m*
uveal uvéal,-e
uveitis uvéite *f*

V

vaccinate, to vacciner
vaccination vaccination *f*
vaccination certificate certificat *m* de vaccination
vaccinaton record carnet *m* de vaccination
vaccine vaccin *m*
vagina vagin *m*
vaginal vaginal,-e
vaginal fornix fornix *m* du vagin
vaginal prolapse prolapsus *m* vaginal
vaginitis vaginite *f*
valve valvule *f*
varicocele varicocèle *f*
variety variété *f*
vascular groove rainure *f* vasculaire
vascularitis vascularite *f*
vaseline™ vaseline™ *f*
vegetable légume *m*
vegetable foods aliments *mpl* végétaux
vegetarian diet régime *m* végétarien
vein veine *f*
vena cava inferior veine *f* cave inférieure
vena cava superior veine *f* cave supérieure
venom venin *m*
ventilation ventilation *f*
ventral surface surface *f* ventrale
vertebra vertèbre *f*
vertebra vertébre *m*
vertebral artery artère *f* vertébrale
vertebrate vertébré *m*
vertical external ear canal conduit *m* auditif externe vertical
vertigo vertige *m*
vestibular syndrome syndrome *m* vestibulaire
vestibular system système *m* vestibulaire
vet/veterinary vétérinaire *m*
veterinary assistant auxiliaire *m* de santé animale
veterinary care soins *mpl* vétérinaires
veterinary certificate certificat *m* vétérinaire
veterinary examination examen *m* vétérinaire
veterinary surgery cabinet *m* vétérinaire

water

via the rectum par voie *f* rectale
villosity villosité *f*
violent brutal,-e
violent injury blessure *f* brutale
viral infection infection *f* virale
virus virus *m*
viscera viscère *m*
viscera viscères *mpl*
visceral visceral,-e
vision vision *f*
vitality vitalité *f*
vitamin enriched/with added vitamins vitaminé,-e
vitiligo vitiligo *m*
vitreous humour humeur *f* vitreuse
vomit, to vomir
vomiting vomissement *m*
voracious vorace
vulva vulve *f*
vulvitis vulvite *f*

W

waiting room salle *f* d'attente
walk, to marcher
wall (stomach etc) paroi *m*
walnut noix *m*
warble, to ramager
warfarin warfarine *f*
warm up, to échauffer
warning sign signe *m* avant-coureur
warning signs signes *mpl* prémonitoires
wart verrue *f*
washing toilette *f*
washing out lavage *m*
wasp sting piqûre *f* de guêpe
wasteful gaspilleur/gaspilleuse
wasting disease maladie *f* de langeur
water eau *f*

water bottle biberon *m*
water container abreuvoir *m*
waterproof étanche
watery stools selles *fpl* humides
wax cire *f*
weakness faiblesse *f*
wean, to sevrer
weaning sevrage *m*
weaving tic *m* de l'ours
weigh, to peser
weight poids *m*
welfare bien-être *m*
well looked after bien soigné,-e
wellbeing bien-être *m*
wet nose truffe *f* humide
wet tail maladie *f* de la queue mouillée
wheat blé *m*
wheezing wheezing *m*
whelp, to mettre bas
whelp, to mettre en bas
when to use (drugs etc) indications *fpl* thérapeutiques
whinny, to hennir
whinnying hennisement *m*
whipworm trichure *f*
whiskers moustaches *fpl*
whistling sifflement *m*
white blood cells globules *mpl* blancs
white line ligne *f* blanche
wild plant plante *f* sauvage
wind souffle *m*
windpipe trachée *f*
wing aile *f*
wing tip pointe *f* d'aile
wingspan envergure *f*
winter coat robe *f* d'hiver
winter plumage plumage *m* d'hiver
with eyes closed aux yeux *mpl* fermés
with eyes open aux yeux *mpl* ouverts
with retained testicles cryptorchidie *m*
wither pad tapis *m* de garrot
withers garrot *m*

wood shavings copeaux *mpl* de bois
work horse cheval de travail *m*
working fonctionnel/ fonctionnelle
worm, to vermifuger
worming vermifugation *f*
worming product vermifuge *m*
worms vers *mpl*
wound blessure *f*
wound plaie *f*
wounded blessé,-e
wrist carpe *m*
wrist poignet *m*

X,Y,Z

x-ray radio *f*
yap, to clabauder
yap, to japper
yearling yearling *m*
yeast tablets comprimés *mpl* de levure
yellow fat disease maladie *f* de la graisse jaune
yelp, to japper
yersinial infection yersiniose *f*
yew if *m*
young mice souriceaux *mpl*
zinc zinc *m*
zoonosis zoonose *f*
zygote zygote

FRENCH-ENGLISH

A

abandon *m* **des jeunes** abandonning of the litter
abattement *m* depression
abattement *m* exhaustion
abcès *m* abcess
abdomen *m* abdomen
abdominal,-e abdominal
abduction *f* abduction
abeille *f* bee
aberrant,-e *adj* aberrant
aberration *f* aberration
aberration *f* **chromosomique** chromosomic aberration
abreuver *v* provide water, to (for animal); **s'abreuver** drink, to (animal)
abreuvoir *m* water container
abreuvoir *m* **automatique** automatic waterer
abri *m* shelter
absorbant,-e *adj* absorbent
acares *mpl* mites
acariens *mpl* **auriculaires** ear mites
accident *m* accident
accident *m* **de la circulation** road traffic accident
accident *m* **vasculaire cérébral (abb AVC)** cerebral vascular accident CVA
accouchement *m* **déclenché** induced labour
accouplement *m* mating
accueil *m* reception
acétabulum *m* acetabulum
achalasie *f* achalasia
acide *m* **aminé** amino acid
acide *m* **arachidonique** arachidonic acid
acide *m* **folique** folic acid
acide *m* **linoléïque** linoleic acid
acide *m* **urique** uric acid
acides *mpl* **gras essentiels** essential fatty acids
acidose *f* acidosis
acné *f* acne
aconit *m* monkshood

112

acromégalie *f* acromegaly
acromégalie *f* acromegalia
activité *f* **réduite** reduced activity
acuité *f* acuity, acuteness
acupuncture *f* acupuncture
addiction *f* addiction
adénite *f* adenitis
adénome *m* adenoma
adénome *m* **de la prostate** prostate gland enlargement
adhérence *f* adhesion
adrénaline *f* adrenaline
adulte *m* adult
affaissement *m* sinking
affection *f* affection; ailment
affection *f* **héréditaire** hereditary trait
affections *fpl* **nerveuses** nervous afflictions
agalactie *f* agalactia
âge *m* age
âge *m* **idéal de reproduction** best age for reproduction
agglutination *f* agglutination
agglutiner *v* agglutinate, to
agglutinine *f* agglutinin
agiter (s') *v* be disturbed, to
agiter (s') *v* be restless, to
agressif/agressive *adj* aggressive
aigu, aiguë *adj* acute
aiguiser ses griffes *v* sharpen its claws, to
aile *f* wing
aile *f* **bâtarde** bastard wing
aine *f* groin
albinisme *m* albinism
albinos *adj* albino
albumine *f* albumin
albuminurie *f* albuminuria
alcalose *f* alkalosis
alcool *m* alcohol
alcool *m* **à 90** surgical spirit
alcool *m* **absolu** pure alcohol
aliment *m* **humide** moist food
aliment *m* **industriel** proprietary food
alimentation *f* feed

alimentation *f* **déséquilibrée** unbalanced diet
alimentation *f* **light** reduced calorie food
alimentation *f* **trop riche** too rich a diet
aliments *mpl* **adaptés à** suitable food for
aliments *mpl* **tout prêts** ready-made food
aliments *mpl* **végétaux** vegetable foods
allaitement *m* **artificiel** artificial feeding
aller au petit gallop *v* canter, to
allergène *m* allergen
allergie *f* allergy
allergie *f* **alimentaire** food allergy
allergie *f* **cutanée** skin allergy
allergie *f* **respiratoire** respiratory allergy
allergique à allergic, to
allongement *m* **du voile du palais** elongated soft palate
alopécie *f* alopecia
alopécie *f* **endocrinienne féline** feline endocrine alopecia
alula *m* alula
alvéolite *f* **pulmonaire** alveolitis of the lungs
amaigrir slim, to
amaigrissé,-e emaciated
amaigrissement *m* loss of weight
amaigrissement *m* emaciation
amniotique amniotic
amphétamine *f* amphetamine
ampoule *f* ampulla
ampoule *f* **rectale** rectal ampulla
amputation *f* amputation
amygdalite *f* tonsillitis
amyloïdose *f* amyloidosis
anabolisant *m* anabolic steroid
anabolisant *m* **stéroïdien** anabolic steroid
anabolisme *m* anabolism
analgésique *m* analgesic
analyse *f* analysis
analyse *f* **de sang** blood test
analyse *f* **de selles** feacal analysis
analyse *f* **d'urine** urine analysis
anaphylaxie *f* anaphylaxia
anasthésie *f* anaesthesia
anasthésie *f* **générale** general anaesthetic

anasthésie *f* **locale** local anaesthetic
âne *m* donkey
anémie *f* anaemia
anémie *f* **aplasique** aplastic anaemia
anémie *f* **aplastique** aplastic anaemia
anémie *f* **infectieuse équine** equine infectious anaemia
anémie *f* **infectieuse féline** feline infectious anaemia
anémie *f* **pernicieuse** pernicious anaemia
anémie *f* **pernicieuse progressive** progressive pernicious anaemia
anémique anaemic
anérobique anaerobic
anesthésier anaesthetize, to
anesthésique *m* anaesthetic
anévrisme *m* aneurism
angine *f* tonsillitis
angine *f* **de poitrine** angina
angiome *m* angioma
animal *m* **de compagnie** pet
ankyloblépharon *m* ankyloblepharon
ankylostamiase *f* ankylostomiasis
ankylostamiase *f* uncinariasis
ankylostome *f* hookworm
ankylostomose *f* hookworm disease
anneau *m* **inguinal profond** deep inguinal ring
anneau *m* **inguinal superficiel** superficial inguinal ring
anoestrus *m* anœstrus
anomalie *f* anomaly
anomalie *f* **de l'œil du colley** collie eye anomaly CEA
anorexie *f* anorexia
anorexique anorexic
anoure anoura
anoxie *f* anoxia
antalgique analgesic
antalgique painkilling
antibiotique *m* antibiotic
anticancéreux/anticancéreuse anticancer
anticancéreux/anticancéreuse antineoplastic
anticoagulant *m* anticoagulant
anticoagulant,-e anticoagulant
anticorps *mpl* antibodies
antidiarrhéique *m* antidiarrheic

antidote *m* antidote
antifongique antifungal
antigel *m* antifreeze
antigène *m* antigène m
antigénique antigenic
antihelmintique *m* anthelmintic
antihistaminique *m* antihistaminic
antihistaminique *m* antihistamine
anti-inflammatoire anti-inflammatory
antiparasitaire *m* insecticide
antipyrétique antipyretic
antiseptique *m* antiseptic
antisérum *m* antiserum
antitoxine *f* anti-toxin
antitoxique antitoxic
antitussif/antitussive antitussive
antiviral,-e antiviral
antivomatif *m* antiemetic
anurie *f* anuresis
anurie *f* anuria
anus *m* anus
anxiété *f* anxiety
aorte *f* aorta
aorte *f* **abdominale** abdominal aorta
aorte *f* **thoracique** thoracic aorta
aoûats *mpl* chiggers; harvest mites
apathie *f* apathy
aphte *m* mouth ulcer
aplasie *f* **médullaire** medullary aplasia
aplomb *m* balance
apoplexie *f* apoplexy, stroke
appareil *m* **digestif** digestive system
appareil *m* **locomoteur** motor system
appareil *m* **respiratoire** respiratory system/tract
appât *m* **empoisoné** poisoned bait
appétence *f* appetency
appliquer apply, to
apprentissage *m* **de la propreté** toilet training
apprivoisé,-e tame
apprivoisé,-e domesticated
apprivoiser tame, to

116

approprié,-e appropriate
araignée *f* venimeuse poisonous spider
arcade *f* sourcilière arch of the eyebrow
arracher extract, to (tooth etc)
arracher pull out, to
arrêt *m* du cœur heart failure
arrêt *m* respiratoire respiratory failure
artère *f* artery
artère *f* axillaire axillary artery
artère *f* carotide carotid artery
artère *f* cervicale profonde profound cervical artery
artère *f* cervicale superficielle superficial cervical artery
artère *f* iliaque iliac artery
artère *f* iliaque externe external iliac artery
artère *f* iliaque interne internal iliac artery
artère *f* pulmonaire pulmonary artery
artère *f* pulmonaire droite right pulmonary artery
artère *f* pulmonaire gauche left pulmonary artery
artère *f* thoracique externe external thoracic artery
artère *f* thoracique interne internal thoracic artery
artère *f* tibiale caudale caudal tibial artery
artére *f* tibiale crâniale cranial tibial artery
artère *f* vertébrale vertebral artery
artériosclérose *f* arterioscelerosis
artérite *f* arteritis
arthrite *f* arthritis
arthrite *f* septique septic arthritis
arthrocentèse *f* arthrocentisis
Arthropodes *mpl* Arthropoda
arthrose *f* non-inflammatory arthritis
arthrose *f* de la hanche osteo-arthritis of the hip
arthrose *f* primaire primary osteoarthritis
arthrose *f* secondaire secondary arthritis
articulation *f* joint
articulation *f* de la hanche hip joint
articulation *f* de l'épaule shoulder joint
articulation *f* du boulet fetlock joint
articulation *f* du coude elbow joint
articulation *f* du genou stifle joint
articulation *f* du pied coffin joint
arythmie *f* cardiaque cardiac arrythmia

ascaride *m* ascarid
ascaride *m* roundworm
ascaris *m* **du chat** toxocara cati
ascaris *m* **du chien** toxocara canis
ascendance *f* ancestry
ascite *f* ascites
aspergillose *f* aspergillosis
asphyxie *f* asphyxia
aspirer le pus draw the pus, to
assimilable easily assimilated
assouplissement *m* suppling
assurance *f* insurance
assurance *m* **animaux de compagnie** pet insurance
astasie-abasie *f* astasia-abasia
asthénie *f* asthenia
asthénique asthenic
asthme *m* asthma
astringent astringent
ataxie *f* ataxia
ataxie *f* **locomotrice** locomotor ataxia
ataxique ataxic
atélectasie *f* atelectasis
atlas *m* atlas
atopie *f* atopy
atrophie *f* atrophy
atrophie *f* **rétinienne** retinal atrophy
atrophier atrophy, to
attaque *f* **cérébrale** stroke
atteindre affect, to; reach, to
atteint,-e affected
attraper catch, to
au pré at grass
aubiose *m* auboise
audition *f* hearing
audition *f* **abîmée** poor hearing
auge *f* manger
augmentation *f* **de la soif** increasing thirst
augmentation *f* **de la température** increasing temperature
augmenter increase, to
ausculter sound (chest etc), to
autogène autogenous

autogène autogenic
auto-immunité *f* auto-immunity
autolyse *f* autolysis
autonome self-sufficient
autopsie *f* necropsy
autopsie *f* post-mortem
autotoxine *f* autotoxin
aux yeux *mpl* **fermés** with eyes closed
aux yeux *mpl* **ouverts** with eyes open
auxiliaire *m* **de santé animale** veterinary assistant
avaler swallow, to
avant-bras *m* forearm
avant-main *f* forehand
aveugle blind
avoir chaud be hot, to
avoir de la fièvre run a temperature, to
avoir de la fièvre have a high temperature, to
avoir froid be cold, to
avoir mal be in pain, to
avoir peur be afraid/frightened, to
avoir/faire une rechute have a relapse, to
avortement *m* abortion
avulsion *f* **dentaire** tooth extraction
axillaires *fpl* axillaries
azoospermatisme *m* azoospermatism
azoospermie *f* azoospermia

B

babésiose *f* babesiosis
babinebalanite *f* balanitis
babines *fpl* flews
bac *m* **à litière** litter tray
bacille *m* bacillus
bactéries *fpl* bacteria
bague *f* **d'identification** identity ring

baigner bath, to
baignoire *f* bath
bain *m* bath
baisser la température lower the temperature, to
bajoue *f* jowl
bajoues *fpl* cheek pouches
bajoues *fpl* **collées** impacted pouches
balano-posthite *f* balanopostitis
balle *f* **de foin** hay bale
balloné,-e swollen
ballonements *mpl* bloating
bandage *m* **adhésif** self-adhesive bandage
bande *f* **adhésive** adhesive bandage
bande *f* **cranienne** median crown stripe
bande *f* **de repos** stable bandage
bande *f* **de travail** exercise bandage
bande *f* **de travail** leg bandage
bande *f* **Velpeau** crepe bandage
bandeau *m* **de la tête** lateral crown stripe
bandeau *m* **sur l'œil** eye-stripe
banque *f* **de sperme** sperm bank
barbe *f* chin groove
barbelure *f* awn (barb)
barre *f* bar
barres *fpl* **alaires** covert bars
bartonellose cat scratch disease
base *f* **de la queue** dock of tail
base *f* **de la queue** set on of tail
bassin *m* pelvis
bâtard *m* mongrel
bâtonnet *m* **de coton** cotton bud
baver drool, to
baver dribble, to
béant,-e gaping
bébé *m* **furet** kit (ferret)
bec *m* beak, bill
bec-de lièvre *m* harelip
belladone *f* nightshade
bénin, bénigne benign
besoins *mpl* **nutritionnels** nutritional needs
béta-carotène *m* beta-carotene

betterave *f* **à sucre** sugar beet
biberon *m* water bottle
bicoloré,-e bicoloured
bien soigné,-e well looked after
bien-être *m* welfare
bien-être *m* wellbeing
bilan *m* assessment
bilan *m* **de santé** health check
bilan *m* **sanguin** blood check
bile *f* bile
biliverdine *f* biliverdin
biopsie *f* biopsy
bistouri *m* lance
blé *m* wheat
blépharite *f* blepharitis
blessé,-e injured
blessé,-e wounded
blesser injure, to
blesser make sore, to
blesser (se) injure oneself, to
blesser (se) hurt oneself, to
blessure *f* wound
blessure *f* injury
blessure *f* **brutale** violent injury
blessures *fpl* **aux yeux** eye injuries
blocage *m* blockage
boire drink, to
boisson drink
boîte *f* **de voyage** travelling box
boîter limp, to
boiterie *f* lameness
bonne santé *f* good health
borréliose *f* borreliosis
bosse *f* lump
botter kick, to
bottes *fpl* **de canon** brushing boots
bouche *f* mouth
bouché,-e de cire full of wax
bouche-à-bouche *m* mouth to mouth resuscitation
bouchon *m* **de cire** earwax
boule *f* **de poil** fur ball

boulet *m* fetlock
bourgeonnement *m* **d'une plaie** granulation tissue
bourrelet *m* **périoplique** perioplic ring
bourrelet *m* **principal** coronary corium
bourrelet *m* **principal** coronary body
bouton *m* **d'acné** acne (spot)
bouton *m* **d'or** buttercup
box *m* loosebox
bradycardie *f* bradycardia
bradycardique bradycardiac
bradyrythmie *f* bradycardia
bras *m* **supérieur** upper arm
bréchet *m* brisket
bride *f* bridle
bride *f* **à filet** snaffle bit
brider un cheval bridle a horse, to
brochage *m* pinning (bone etc)
bronche *f* bronchus
bronche *f* **droite** right bronchus
bronche *f* **gauche** left bronchus
bronchiolite *f* bronchiolitis
bronchite *f* brochitis
broncho-pneumonie *f* bronchopneumonia
brossage *m* brushing
brossage *m* **regulier** regular brushing
brosser brush, to
brosser les dents brush the teeth, to
brouter graze, to
brucellose *f* brucellosis
bruits *mpl* **cardiaques** heart murmur
brûlant,-e burning
brûlure *f* burn
brutal,-e sudden
brutal,-e violent
bruyant,-e noisy
buis *m* box (plant)

C

cabinet *m* consulting room
cabinet *m* surgery (place)
cabinet *m* **vétérinaire** veterinary surgery
cabrer rear up, to
cabrer (se) rear, to
cacahuètes *fpl* peanuts
cacatoès *m* cockatoo
cachexie *f* cachexia
caecum *m* caecum
cage *f* cage
cage *f* **thoracique** ribcage
caillot *m* clot
caillot *m* **sanguin** blood clot
caisse *f* **de transport** carrying case
calcanéum *m* calcaneus
calcémie *f* calcemia
calcium *m* calcium
calcul *m* **biliaire** gall stone
calcul *m* **rénal** kidney stones
calculs *mpl* stones
cale *f* **en plastique** plastic wedge
calicivirose *f* feline calicivirus
callosité *f* callus
calmant *m* **analgésique** painkiller
calmant *m* **analgésique** analgesic
cancer *m* cancer
cancer *m* **de la prostate** prostate cancer
cancéreux/cancéreuse cancerous
cancérigène carcinogenic
cancériser (se) become cancerous
cancérogène carcinogenic
Candida albicans Candida albicans
candidose *f* candida
canin,-e *adj* canine
canine *f* canine tooth
cannabalisme *m* cannabilism
canon *m* cannon bone
canon *m* **antérieur** forecannon

canon *m* **postérieur** hind-cannon
capelet *m* capped hock
captivité: en captivité in captivity
carcinome *m* carcinoma
carcinome *m* **squameux** squamous cell carcinoma
cardiomyopathie *f* cardiomyopathy
cardiomyopathie *f* **dilatée** dilated cardiomyopathy
cardique cardiac
cardite *f* carditis
carence *f* deficiency
carence *f* **de** lack of
carence *f* **de thiamine** thiamin deficiency
carence *f* **en** lack of; deficiency of
caresse *f* caress
caresser stroke, to
carie *f* tooth decay
carnet *m* **de santé** health record
carnet *m* **de vaccination** vaccinaton record
carnivore carnivorous
carnivore *m* carnivore
carpe *m* carpus
carpe *m* wrist
cartilage *m* cartilage
cartilage *m* **articulaire** articular cartilage
casque *m* **protecteur** hard hat
cassé,-e broken
cassure *f* **du nez** stop
castration *f* castration
castré,-e castrated
castré,-e spayed
castrer geld, to
castrer spay, to
catabolisme *m* catabolism
cataplasme *m* poultice
cataracte *f* cataract
catarrhal,-e catarrhal
catarrhe *m* catarrh
cathétérisme *m* catheterization
caudal,-e caudal
caudectomie *f* docking of the tail
cautère *m* cautery

cautérisation *f* cauterisation
cautériser cauterise, to
cavalier *m* rider
cavité *f* cavity
cavité *f* **abdominale** abdominal cavity
cavité *f* **buccale** oral cavity
cavité *f* **nasale** nasal cavity
cavité *f* **pelvienne** pelvic cavity
cavité *f* **péricardique** pericardal cavity
cavité *f* **péritoneale** peritoneal cavity
cavité *f* **pleurale** pleural cavity
cavité *f* **thoracique** thoracic cavity
cécité *f* blindness
cellule *f* cell
cellulite *f* cellulitis
cellulles *fpl* **cancérisées** cancerous cells
cément *m* **(dent)** cement (tooth)
cercle *m* **orbital** eye ring
céréales *fpl* cereals
cérébral,-e cerebral
cérébro-spinal,-e cerebrospinal
cerf *m* deer
certificat *m* **d'ascendence** pedigree
certificat *m* **de vaccination** vaccination certificate
certificat *m* **vétérinaire** veterinary certificate
cérumen *m* earwax
cerveau *m* brain
cervelet *m* cerebellum
césarienne *f* caesarean section
Cestodes *mpl* Cestoda
chair *f* **feuilletée** sensitive laminae
chalazion *m* chalazion
chaleur: en chaleur calling
chaleur: en chaleur in season
chaleur: en chaleur on heat
chambre *f* **antérieure de l'œil** anterior chamber of the eye
chambre *f* **postérieure de l'œil** posterior chamber of the eye
champ *m* **visuel** field of view
chanfrein *m* muzzle
chanfrein *m* nose
chanter sing, to

chondrodystrophie

charbon *m* anthrax
charbon *m* **de bois** charcoal
chasseur *m* hunter
chat *m*; **chatte** *f* cat
châtaigne *f* chestnut
chaton *m* kitten
châtré,-e neutered
chatte *f* queen
chaud,-e hot
chauffage *m* **de tendon** tenosynovitis
cheilite *f* cheilitis
chemise *f* **de paddock** paddock sheet
chémosis *m* chemosis
chenil *m* kennel
cheval de travail *m* work horse
cheval *m* horse
cheval *m* **difficile** unruly horse
cheville *f* ankle
chevreuil *m* deer
cheyletiellose *f* cheyletiella infection
chien *m*; **chienne** *f* dog; bitch
chien *m* **de berger** sheep dog
chien *m* **de chasse** gun dog
chien *m* **de chasse** hunting dog
chien *m* **de garde** guard dog
chien *m* **rapporteur** retriever
chienne *f* bitch
chiens *mpl* **d'appartement** toy dogs
chiens *mpl* **de grand race** large breed dogs
chiens *mpl* **de petite taille** small dogs
chiffon *m* **"cactus"** "cactus" cloth
chiot *m* puppy
chirurgie *f* surgery, operation
chlamydiose *f* feline chlamydial infection
chlore *m* chlorine
choc *m* shock
choc *m* **anaphylactique** anaphylactic shock
cholécystite *f* cholecystitis
choline *f* choline
chondrodysplasie *f* chondrodysplasia
chondrodystrophie *f* chondrodysplasia

chorée *f* chorea
chorio-méningite *f* choriomeningitis
chorion *m* **de la paroi** laminar corium
choroïde *f* choroid
chromosome *m* chromosome
chronique chronic
chute *f* fall
chute *f* **de plumes** feather loss
chylothorax chylothorax
cicatrice *f* scar
cicatrisation *f* healing (of wound etc)
ciguë *f* hemlock
cil *m* eyelash
cimetière *m* **animalier** pet cemetery
circulation *f* circulation
circumanalomes *mpl* nal adenomata
cire *f* wax
cirrhose *f* cirrhosis
ciseaux *mpl* scissors
clabauder yap, to
claquage *m* **de tendon** tendon bow
claquage *m* **musculaire** pulled muscle
claudication *f* limp
clavicule *f* collarbone
cloaque *m* cloaca
cloches *fpl* overreach boots
clone *m* clone
clou *m* **de rue** puncture wound
coagulant *m* coagulant
coagulation *f* coagulation
cob *m* cob
coccidiose *f* coccidiosis
cochléaire cochlear
cochon *m* **d'inde** guinea pig
cœur *m* heart
coin *m* **(dent)** corner (teeth)
coire *f* dock
coït *m* coitus
col *m* **d'utérus** cervix
colchique *m* meadow saffron
colibacillose *f* colibacillosis

conduit auditif

colique *f* colic
colique *f* néphrétique renal colic
coliques *fpl* de plomb lead poisoning colic
colite *f* colitis
collapsus *m* collapse
collapsus *m* tracheal collapsed trachea
collerette *f* Elizabethan collar
collier *m* anti-puces flea collar
collier *m* de poitrine breastplate
collyre *m* eye drops
collyre *m* eye lotion
côlon *m* colon
côlon *m* descendant descending colon
côlon *m* ventral droit right ventral colon
côlon *m* ventral gauche left ventral colon
colonne vertébrale *f* spinal cord
colonne vertébrale *f* spine
colostomie *f* colostomy
colostrum *m* colostrum
colprocèle *m* colprocele
comateux/comateuse comatose
commissure *f* de la bouche corner of mouth
commotion *f* concussion
commotion *f* cérébrale concussion
communication *f* communication
complément *m* alimentaire food supplement
complexe granulome *m* eosinophilique felin feline rodent ulcer
complications *fpl* complications
comportement *m* behaviour
comportement *m* agressif aggressive behaviour
comporter (se) behave, to
composition *f* ingredients
compresse *f* compress
compresse *f* désinfectante antiseptic compress
comprimé *m* pill
comprimés *mpl* de levure yeast tablets
compte-gouttes *m* dropper
concentré *m* concentrate (food)
concentrés *mpl* concentrates
conception *f* conception
conduit *m* auditif externe horizontal horizontal external ear canal

128

conduit *m* auditif externe vertical vertical external ear canal
conduit *m* lacrymal tear duct
conduit *m* naso-lacrymal nasolacrimal duct
conduits *mpl* lachrymaux lachrymal ducts
conduits *mpl* lachrymaux lachrymatory ducts
confusion *f* confusion
congénital,-e congenital
congestion *f* congestion
conjonctivite *f* conjunctivitis
constant,-e constant
constipation *f* constipation
constipé,-e constipated
consultation *f* consultation
contagieux/contagieuse contagious
contagion *f* contagion
contraction *f* contraction
contre-indication *f* contraindication
contrôle *m* du cheval control of the horse
contrôler control, to
contusion *f* bruise
convulsion *f* convulsion
coopératif/coopérative cooperative
copeaux *mpl* de bois wood shavings
coprophagie *f* coprophagy
cor *m* corn (on foot)
cordon *m* médullaire spinal cord
cordon *m* ombilical umbilical cord
corne *f* hoof horn
cornée *f* cornea
corps *m* body
corps *m* ciliaire ciliary body
corps *m* étranger foreign body
corrosif/corrosive corrosive
cortex *m* cérébral cerebral cortex
corticostéroïdes *mpl* corticosteroids
corticothérapie *f* corticotherapy
cortisone *f* cortisone
coryza *m* coryza, cold in the head
côte *f* rib
côté *m* droite right side
côté *m* gauche left side

crevasser

coton *m* cotton wool
cou *m* neck
couche *f* **cornée** hard skin
coude *m* elbow
couiner squeal, to
couler run, to (of eyes etc)
coup *m* **de chaleur** heat stroke
coup *m* **de soleil** sun burn
coupe *f* **des ongles** nail clipping
couper cut, to
couplement *m* **consanguin** inbreeding
coupler (se) mate, to
coup-ongle *m* nail-clipper
courants *mpl* **d'air** draughts
couronne *f* coronet
coussinet *m* pad
coussinet *m* **carpien** carpal/stopper pad
coussinet *m* **déchiré** cut pad
coussinet *m* **de l'ergot** dew pad
coussinet *m* **digité** digital pad
coussinet *m* **métacarpien** metacarpal pad
coussinet *m* **métatarsien** metatarsal pad
coussinet *m* **palmaire** metacarpal pad
coussinet *m* **plantaire** digital cushion
coussinet *m* **plantaire** metatarsal pad
couteau *m* **de chaleur** sweat scraper
couvaison *f* brooding, incubation
couverture *f* **de refroidissement** cooler
couverture *m* rug
couvertures *fpl* **marginales** outer primary coverts
couvertures *fpl* **moyennes** median coverts
couvertures *fpl* **primaires** primary coverts
crampe *f* cramp
crampon *m* spike
crâne *m* skull
crème *m* cream
crème *m* **antiseptique** antiseptic cream
creux *m* **du jarret** stifle joint
crevasser chap, to
crevasser (se) become chapped, to
crevasser (se) crack, to

130

crinière *f* mane
crinière *f* **rase** hogged mane
crinière *f* **toilettée** trimmed mane
crinière *f* **tressée** plaited mane
crise *f* attack
crise *f* crisis
crise *f* **d'épilepsie** fit
cristallin *m* lens
crochet *m* **à tiques** tick remover
croisé,-e crossed
croisement *m* cross-breeding
croissance *f* growth
croquettes *fpl* dry food
crottin *m* dropping
crottin *m* dung
croupe *f* croup
croupe *f* rump
croupion *m* rump
croûte *f* scab
cryptorchidie *m* with retained testicles
cryptosporidiose *f* cryptosporidiosis
cubitus *m* ulna
cuisse *f* thigh
cuivre *m* copper
cure-pied *m* hoof pick
curer un pied pick out a foot, to
curieux/curieuse inquisitive
cutané,-e cutaneous
cyanose *f* cyanosis
cysthominés *mpl* cysthostomes
cystotomie *f* cystotomy
cytise *f* laburnum

D

dard *m* sting
de race thoroughbred
de race pure breed

déboîter (se) dislocate, to
débourrage *m* breaking in (a horse)
débourrer break in, to
débourrer un cheval break in a horse, to
décédé,-e dead
décharge *f* **électrique** electric shock
déchiré,-e torn
déchirer tear, to
déchirer lacerate, to
déchirer (se) tear, to (muscle etc)
déchirure *f* tear
déchirure *f* laceration
déclencher l'accouchement induce labour, to
décollement *m* **de la rétine** detached retina
décollement *m* **du placenta** detached placenta
décongestif *m* decongestant
décongestionnant *m* decongestant
décongestionner relieve congestion, to
décontamination *f* decontamination
défaut *m* abnormality
défécation *f* defecation
défenses *fpl* **naturelles** natural defences
déféquer defecate, to
déferré,-e unshod
déferrer unshoe, to
déformation *f* **de la queue** malformation of the tail
déformation *f* **osseuse** bone deformity
dégager clear, to (nose, chest etc)
dégâts *mpl* **irréversibles** irreversible damage
dégénération *f* degeneration,
dégénérescence *f* deterioration
dégénérescence *f* **graisseuse** loss of body fat
dégénérescence *f* **maculaire** macula degeneration
déglutition *f* deglutition
dégrader become worse, to
dégrader (se) deteriorate, to
démangéaison *f* itch
démangeasion *f* **persistante** persistant wound
démanger itch, to
démêloir *m* large tooth-comb
demodecie *f* demodetic mange

démodecie *f* demodecia
démodécie *f* **généralisée** generalised mange
démodécie *f* **localisée** localised mange
démodex *m* demodex
dent *f* tooth
dent *f* **de lait** milk tooth
dent *f* **incisive** incisor
dent *f* **permanente** permanent tooth
dentine *f* dentine
dentiste *m* **équin** horse dentist
dents *fpl* **à croissance continue** continually growing teeth
dépendence *f* addiction
dépigmentation *f* **du museau** depigmentation of the muzzle
dépilation *f* loss of hair/fur
dépistage *m* screening
dépister detect, to (disease etc)
déplacer displace, to
déreglement *m* **hormonal** hormonal disturbance
dermaophytes *mpl* dermatophytes
dermatite *f* dermatitis
dermatite *f* **miliare** miliary dermatitis
dermatite *f* **solaire** solar dermatitis
dermatomycose *f* dermatomycosis
dermatophytie *f* dermatophytosis
dermatophytose *f* dermatophytosis
dermatose *f* **prurigineuse** pruriginous dermatosis
dermatoses *fpl* **bactériennes** bacterial dermatosis
derme *m* dermis
dermite *f* dermatitis
dermoïde *m* **cornéen** dermoid of the cornea
désarçonner le cavalier throw the rider, to
déséquilibres *mpl* **hormonaux** imbalance of hormones
déshydraté,-e dehydrated
déshydrater (se) dehydrate, to
désinfectant *m* disinfectant
désinfecter disinfect, to
désintoxication *f* detoxification
désintoxiquer detoxify, to
désobéissance *f* disobedience
désordre *m* disorder
désordres *mpl* **intestinaux** intestinal disorders

desseller unsaddle, to
destructeur/destructrice destructive
détartrage *m* descaling
détente *f* relaxation
deuxième phalange *f* phalanx secunda
développement *m* **osseux** bone growth
développement *m* **osseux** bony enlargement
déviation *f* deviation
déviation *f* displacement
déviation *f* inversion
déviation *f* curvature
diabète *m* diabetes
diabète *m* **insipide** diabetis insipidus
diabète *m* **rénal** renal diabetis
diabète sucré diabetes mellitus
diabétique diabetic
diagnose *f* diagnosis
diagnostic *m* diagnosis
diagnostique diagnostic
diagnostiquer diagnose, to
diagostic *m* **précoce** early diagnosis
dialyse *f* dialysis
diaphragme *m* diaphragm
diarrhée *f* diarrhoea
diathermique *f* diathermy
différenciation *f* **des sexes** distinguishing the sexes
difficile difficult
difficultés *fpl* **pour uriner** difficulty in urinating
difformité *f* **congenitale** congenital deformity
difformité *f* **de la voie nasolacrymale** nasolacrimal duct deformity
digérer digest, to
digestible digestible
digestion *f* digestion
digestion *f* **paresseuse** lazy digestion
digitale *f* foxglove
dilatation-torsion *f* **de l'estomac** bloat
dilitation *f* dilation
dilitation *f* **de l'oreillette droite** dilation of the right atrium cordis
dilitation *f* **de l'oreillette gauche** dilation of the left atrium cordis
dimensions *fpl* **de la cage** cage size
diplégie *f* diplegia

dipylidium caninum *m* dipylidium caninum
dirofilariose *f* dirofilariosis
dislocation *f* dislocation
disloquer (se) dislocate, to
distichiasis *f* distichiasis
diurétique *m* diuretic
diurne diurnal
docteur *m* doctor
donner un bain bath, to
dorsal,-e dorsal
dos *m* back
dos *m* **de mulet** roach back
dos *m* **fortement ensellé** sway back
dossier *m* file
douleur *f* pain
drain *m* drainage tube, drain
drainer drain, to
drip goutte à goutte f
drip *m* **feeding** drip feeding
drogue *f* drug
duodénite *f* duodenitis
duodénum *m* duodenum
dur,-e hard
durée *f* **de gestation** length of pregnancy
dysautonomie *f* **féline** feline dysautonomia
dyslipémie *f* dyslipemia
dyslipidémie *f* dyslipemia
dyspesie *f* indigestion
dysphagie *f* dysphagia
dysplasie *f* dysplasia
dysplasie *f* **de la hanche** hip dysplasia
dyspnée *f* dyspnea
dystocie *f* dystocia
dystrophie *f* **cornéenne** corneal dystrophy
dystrophie *f* **épithéliale** epithelial dystrophy
dysurie *f* dysuria

E

eau *f* water
eau *f* **de Javel** household bleach
eau *f* **oxygénée** hydrogen peroxide
ébouillanté,-e scalded
ébouriffé,-e ruffled
ébrouer (s') snort, to
échantillion *m* specimen (eg of urine)
écharde *f* splinter
échaudure *f* rain scald
échauffement *f* **de la fourchette** thrush
échauffer overheat, to
échauffer warm up, to
échinococcose *f* echinococcosis
échographie *f* scan
éclaircir la crinière thin the mane, to
éclaircir la queue thin the tail, to
éclampsie *f* eclampsia
écorchure *f* abrasion
écoulement *m* **des yeux** runny eyes
écoulement *m* **nasal** nasal discharge
écoulement *m* **vulvaire** discharge from the vulva
écoulements *mpl* discharge
écrasement *m* crushing
ectopie *f* **testiculaire** ectopic testicle
éctopie *f* **uréterale** ureteral ectopia
ectropion *m* ectropion
écuelle *f* food bowl
écume *f* foam
écurie *f* stable
eczéma *m* **faciel** facial eczema
effets *mpl* **non souhaités et gênants** side effects
effets *mpl* **secondaires** side effects
efficacité *f* effectiveness
efficacité *f* efficacy
efflanqué slab-sided
effleurage *m* effleurage
effleurage *m* light massage
électrocardiogramme *m* **ECG** electrocardiogram ECG
électrocardiographie *f* **ECG** electrocardiograph ECG

électrocution *f* electrocution
électroencéphalogramme *m* **EEG** electroencephalogram EEG
électroencéphalographie *f* **EEG** electroencephalogram EEG
électrolytes *mpl* electrolytes
élevage *m* breeding
éleveur *m* breeder
élimination *f* elimination
éliminer eliminate, to
élongation *f* strained/pulled muscle
emaciation *f* emaciation
embolie *f* embolism
embolie *f* **artérielle** arterial embolism
embolie *f* **cérébrale** cerebral embolism
embonpoint *m* plumpness
embrocation *f* embrocation
embryon *m* embryo
embryonnaire embryonic
emétique *m* emetic
emphysème *m* **pulmonaire** pulmonary emphysema
emplâtre *m* cold pack
empoisonnement *m* poisoning
empoisonnement *m* **du sang** blood poisoning
empoisonner poison, to
encéphalite *f* encephalitis
encéphalomyélite *f* encephalomyelitis
encolure *f* neck; crest of neck
encolure *f* **de cerf** ewe neck
encoprésie *f* encopresis
endémie *f* endemic disease
endémique endemic
endocardiose *f* **mitrale** mitral endocardiosis
endocardite *f* endocarditis
endomètre *m* endometrium
endométrite *f* endometritis
endormi,-e asleep
endoscope *m* endoscope
endoscople *f* endoscopy
enflammé,-e inflamed
enflure *f* swelling
enflure *f* **abdominale** abdominal swelling
enfoncement *m* traumatic depression

137

engorgement *m* engorgement
engorgement *m* obstruction
engorger engorge, to
engorger obstruct, to
engoudissement *m* numbness
enlever remove, to
enlever les crottins remove the droppings, to
enlever les ovaries spay, to
ennui *m* boredom
enragé,-e rabid; mad
enrichi,-e de enriched with
enrobé,-e plump
ensellement *m* hollow
entartrement *m* scaling
entérite *f* enteritis
entérite *f* **chronique** chronic enteritis
entérocolite *f* entrocolitis
entérotomie *f* enterotomy
entérotoxémie *f* enterotoxemia
entérovirus *m* enterovirus
entorse *f* sprain
entraînement *m* training
entraîner train, to
entropion *m* entropion
enurèse *f* enuresis
enurésie *f* enuresis
envergure *f* wingspan
enzootique enzootic
enzyme *m* enzyme
épanchement *m* **pleural** pleural effusion
éparvin *m* **calleux** bone spavin
éparvins *mpl* spavins
épaule *f* shoulder
épaule *f* **inclinée** sloping shoulder
épidémie *f* epidemic
épiderme *m* epidermis
epididymite *f* epididymitis
épiglotte *f* epiglottis
épilepsie *f* epilepsy
épilepsie *f* **esentielle** essential epilepsy
épillet *m* burr

épine *f* thorn
epiphora *m* epiphora
epispadias *m* epispadias
epistaxis *f* epistaxis
éponge *f* capped elbow
éponge *f* sponge
épreuve *f* test
épreuve *f* sur/de la descendance progeny testing
éprouver test, to
épuisement *m* exhaustion
épulis *m* epulis
équarrissage *m* knackers yard
équestre equestrian
équidé *m* equine
équilibre *m* balance
équin *adj* equine
équipement *m* equipment
équipement *m* d'écurie stable equipment
équitation *f* equitation
éradication *f* eradication
éradiquer eradicate
ergot *m* dewclaw
érisipèle *m* erysipelas
érosion *f* abrasion
éruption *f* rash
érysipèle *m* erysipelas
érythème *m* erythema
érythocyte *m* erythrocyte
eschare *f* bedsore
espèce *f* species
essentiel/essentielle essential
estomac *m* stomach
estomac *m* fragile sensitive stomach
étalon *m* stallion
étalon *m* qui a fait ses preuves proven stallion/sire
étanche waterproof
éternuement *m* sneeze
éternuements *mpl* sneezing
éternuer sneeze, to
ethylène *m* glycol ethylene glycol
étiologie *f* aetiology

faire l'ablation

étouffement *m* suffocation
étrangler (s') choke, to
être coincé,-e be trapped,to
étrier *m* stirrup
étrille *f* curry comb
étriller curry, to
euthanasie *f* euthanasia
euthanasier put down, to
eutocie *m* eutocia
évanouir (s') faint, to
évoluer evolve, to
évoluer develop, to
évolutif/évolutive progressive
examen *m* **medical** examination
examen *m* **vétérinaire** veterinary examination
exciter excite to
exciter stimulate, to
excreta *m* excreta
excréter excrete, to
excrétion *f* excretion
excroissance *f* excressance
excroissance *f* outgrowth
exercice *m* exercise
expectorant,-e expectorant
externe external
extraction *f* extraction
extraire extract, to (tooth etc)
extrasystole *f* extrasystole

F

facile easy
façon *m* **de manger** eating habits
facture *f* bill (money)
faiblesse *f* weakness
faire (se) mal hurt oneself, to
faire halt halt to
faire l'ablation de take out, to

faire ses dents teethe, to
faire ses nuits sleep through the night, to
faire un examen examine, to
fanon *m* dewlap
faradisation *f* Faradism
fatigue *f* fatigue
fausse-couche *f* miscarriage
fecalome *m* fecaloma
fèces *fpl* faeces
fécond,-e fertile
fécondation *f* fertilisation
fécondé,-e fertilised
féculents *mpl* carbohydrates
félin *adj* feline
femelle *f* female
femelle *f* bitch
femelle *f* **furet** jill
fémoral,-e femoral
fémur *m* thighbone
fémur *m* femur
fémur *m* upper thigh
fendillé,-e chapped
fer *m* iron
fer *m* shoe (horse)
fermenter ferment, to
ferrage *m* shoeing
ferré,-e shod
fers *mpl* à **pince laminée** shoes with rolled toes
fertilité *f* fertility
fesse *f* buttock
feux *mpl* **d'artifice** fireworks
fibre *m* fibre
fibres *m* **alimentaires** dietary fibre
fibrocartilage *m* fibrocartilage
fibrome *m* fibroma
fibrome *m* fibroid
fibrosarcome *m* fibrosarcoma
fibula *m* fibula
fiche *f* form
fiente *m* droppings (of bird)
fièvre fever

frelon

fiévre f aphteuse foot and mouth disease
fiévreux, fiévreuse feverish
fil m de fer barbelé barbed wire
filet m à foin haynet
filière f pelvienne birth canal
fissure f fissure
fistule f fistula
flanc m flank
flexion f flexion
flore f intestinale intestinal flora
fluctuation f hormonale hormonal fluctuation
flux m sanguin blood flow
fœtus m fœtus
foie f liver
foin m artificiel seed hay
foin m du pré meadow hay
follicule m pileux hair follicle
folliculite f folliculitis
fonctionnel/fonctionnelle functional
fonctionnel/fonctionnelle working
fonctionnement m functioning
forgeron m blacksmith
forme: en pleine forme fit
forme f cartiligineuse sidebone
fornix m du vagin vaginal fornix
forte température f hign temperature
fougère f bracken
foulée f stride
fouler (se) sprain, to
fourbure f founder
fourchette f frog (on hoof)
fourmilière f en pince seedy toe
fourni,-e thick
fourrage m roughage
fourreau m sheath
fourrure f fur
fracture f fracture
fracture f incomplète greenstick fracture
fracturé,-e fractured
fragile fragile
frelon m hornet

fréquence *f* **respiratoire** respiratory rate
friandises *fpl* titbits
friandises *fpl* treats
frisson *m* shiver
frissonner shiver, to
froid *m* **aux jambes** cold to the legs
froid,-e cold
froisser (se) un muscle strain a muscle, to
front *m* forehead
frottant contre chafing
fruit *m* fruit
fumier *m* manure
furet *m* ferret
furoncle *m* furuncle
furonculose *f* furonculosis

G

gabarit *m* build
galactorhée *f* galactorrhea
gale *f* mange
gale *f* scabies
gale *f* **auriculaire** auricular scabies
gale *f* **de la tête** feline scabies
galop *m* gallop
gamelle *f* food bowl
Gamgee *m* Gamgee tissue
gamma-globuline *f* gamma globulin
ganache *f* cheek
ganglion *m* ganglion
ganglion *m* **lymphatique** lymph node
ganglions *m* **lymphatiques** lymph glands
gangrène *f* gangrene
gants *mpl* **latex** rubber/latex gloves
garrot *m* garrot
garrot *m* withers
gaspilleur/gaspilleuse wasteful
gastrique gastric

globuline

gastrite *f* gastritis
gastro-entérite *f* gastroenteritis
gastrophile *m* horse bot
gazouiller chirp, to
gelule *f* capsule
gelure *f* frostbite
gencive *f* gum
gencives *fpl* **pâles** pale gums
gène *m* gene
génétique genetic
genou *m* knee
genoux *mpl* **brassicourts** over at the knee
genoux *mpl* **creux** back at the knee
genoux *mpl* **de mouton** calf knees
gerbille *f* gerbil
gésier *m* gizzard
gestation *f* gestation
gestation *f* pregnancy
giardia *m* giardia
giardiose *m* giardiosis
gingivite *f* gingivitis
glande *f* gland
glande *f* **anale** scent gland
glande *f* **de Harder** Harderian gland
glande *f* **lacrymale** lachrymal gland
glande *f* **parathyroïde** parathyroid gland
glande *f* **pituitaire** pituitary gland
glande *f* **sébacée** sebaceous gland
glande *f* **sudoripare** sweat gland
glande *f* **uropygienne** uropygial gland
glandes *fpl* **anales** anal glands
glandes *fpl* **endocrines** endocrine glands
glandes *fpl* **inguinales** inguinal glands
glandes *fpl* **mammaires** mammary glands
glandes *fpl* **salivaires** salivary glands
glands *mpl* acorns
glaucome *m* glaucoma
globule *m* **rouge** erythrocyte
globules *mpl* **blancs** white blood cells
globules *mpl* **rouge** red blood cells
globuline *f* globulin

glomérulonéphrite *f* glomérulonephritis
glossite *f* glossitis
glucose *m* glucose
glycérine *f* glycerine
glycérol *m* glycerine
glycosurie *f* glycosuria
goitre *m* goitre
gonade *f* gonad
gonflé,-e distended
gonflé,-e swollen
gonflement *m* distension
gonflement *m* swelling
gonflements *mpl* **sous-cutanés** subcutaneous swellings
gonfler swell, to
gorge *f* throat
gosier *m* throatlash
gourme *f* impetigo
gourme *f* strangles
goût *m* taste
goutte *f* drop
goutte *f* gout
gouttes *fpl* **pour le nez** nosedrops
gouttes *fpl* **pour les oreilles** ear drops
gouttes *fpl* **pour les yeux** eyedrops
gouttière *f* **cutigérale** coronary groove
graines *fpl* **de tournesol** sunflower seeds
graines *mpl* cereals
grand sésamoïde *m* proximal sesamoid
grands strongles *mpl* large strongyles
grand ver *m* **rouge** large red worm
grand,-e large
grandes couvertures *fpl* greater coverts
granules *mpl* à **cheveaux** horse nuts
granulocyte *m* granulocyte
granulome *m* granuloma
grasset *m* stifle
gravide pregnant
gravillons *mpl* grit
grelotter de shiver with (shock etc), to
griffe *f* claw
griffes *fpl* **longues** long claws

145

griffoir *m* scratching post
griffure *f* scratch
grignoter nibble, to
grimper climb, to
grincer les dents grind the teeth, to
grippe *f* **aviare** avian flu; bird flu
grippe *f* **équine** equine influenza
grognement *m* grunting
grossesse *f* **nerveuse** false pregnancy
grossesse *f* **nerveuse** phantom pregnancy
grosseur *f* lump
grossir put on weight, to
guêpe *f* wasp
guérir cure, to
guérison *f* recovery
guérison *f* healing
guérissable curable
guêtres *fpl* **de tendon** tendon boots
guêtres *fpl* **de voyage** travelling boots
gueule *f* mouth
guide *f* rein
gynécomastie *f* gynaecomastia

H

habitudes *fpl* **alimentaires** eating habits
habituel/habituelle constant
habronémose *f* **cutanée** sweet itch
hack *m* hack
haie *f* hedge
haleine *f* breath
halètement *m* panting
haleter pant, to
halitose *f* bad breath
hamster *m* hamster
haras *m* stud farm
haras *m* **national** national stud farm
harde *f* herd
harnais *m* harness

harnais *m* **de sécurité** safety harnass
hautement digestible highly digestible
Helicobacter pylori Campylobacter pylori
hémaglobinurie *f* haemoglobinuria
hémarthrose *f* haemarthrosis
hématémèse *f* haematemesis
hématie *f* erythrocyte
hématologie *f* haematology
hématoma *m* haematoma
hématome *m* **auriculaire** aural haematoma
hématurie *f* haematuria
hemeralopie *f* night blindness
hémobartonellose *f* **féline** feline hemobartonellosis
hémoglobine *f* haemoglobin
hémolyse *f* haemolysis
hémoperitoine *m* haemoperitoneum
hémophilie *f* haemophilia
hémoptysie *f* haemoptysis
hémorragie *f* haemorrhage
hémorragie *f* **externe** external bleeding
hémorragie *f* **interne** internal bleeding
hémostase *f* haemostasis
hennir neigh, to
hennir whinny, to
hennisement *m* whinnying
hennissement *m* neighing
héparine *f* heparin
hépatite *f* hepatitis
hépatite *f* **contagieuse** infectious canine hepatitis
herbe *f* grass
herbe *f* **aux chats** cat nip
herbe *f* **aux chats** cat mint
herbe *m* **en sac plastique** haylage
herbivore herbivorous
hérédité *f* heredity
hermaphrodisme *m* hermaphrodism
hernie *f* hernia
hernie *f* **étranglée** strangulated hernia
hernie *f* **locale** slipped disc
hernie *f* **ombilicale** umbilical hernia
herpès *m* herpes

147

herpèsvirus *m* **canin** canine herpes virus
hibernation *f* hibernation
hiberner hibernate, to
histiocytome *m* histiocytoma
hongre *m* gelding
hormone *m* hormone
huile *f* oil
huile *f* **de paraffine** liquid paraffin
huile *f* **de ricin** castor oil
humérus *m* humerus
humeur *f* **aqueuse** aqueous humour
humeur *f* **vitreuse** vitreous humour
humide damp
humidité *f* dampness
hurler howl, to
hydrocèle *f* hydrocele
hydronéphrose *f* hydronephrosis
hydrothérapie *f* hydrotherapy
hygiène *f* hygiene
hygiène *f* **buccale** oral hygiene
hygroma *m* bursitis
hypercalcémie *f* hypercalcemia
hyperfonctionnement *m* **des surrénales** overactive adrenal glands
hyperlipémie *f* hyperlipaemia
hyperlipidémie *f* hyperlipaemia
hyperplasie *f* hyperplasia
hypertension *f* **artérielle** hypertension
hyperthermie *f* hyperthermia
hyperthyroïdie *f* hyperthyroidism
hyperthyroïdisme *m* hyperthyroidism
hypertrophie *f* hypertrophy
hypertrophie *f* **mammaire** mammary hypertrophy
hypervitaminose *f* hypervitaminosis
hypocalcémie *f* hypogcalcemia
hypofonctionnement *m* **des   surrénales** underactive adrenal glands
hypoglycémie *f* hypoglycemia
hypokaliémie *f* hypokalemia
hypoplasie *f* hypoplasia
hypoplasie *f* **cérébelleuse congenitale** congenital cerebellar
    hypoplasis
hypoplasie *f* **génitale** genital hypoplasia

hypospadias *m* hypospadias
hypothermie *f* hypothermia
hypothyroïdie *f* hypothyroidism
hypoxie *f* hypoxia
hystérectomie *f* hysterectomy

I

iatrogène iatrogenic
iatrogénique iatrogenic
ichtyose *f* ichtyosis
ictère *m* jaundice
idiopathique idiopathic
if *m* yew
iléite *f* **proliférative** ileitus
ileus *m* ileus
iliaque iliac
immobiliser immobilise, to
immunisation *f* immunisation
immunisation *f* **contre** immunisation against
immunité *f* immunity
immunité *f* **acquise** acquired immunity
immunodéficience *f* **féline** feline immunodeficiency virus
imperforation *f* **des voies lacrymales** unperforated tear ducts
impétigo *m* impetigo
implant *m* **contaceptif** contraceptive implant
imprévisible unpredictable
inappétence *f* inappetence
incendie *f* fire
incinération *f* cremation
inciser cut, to
incision *f* cut
incisive *f* incisor
incisive *f* **inférieure** lower incisor
incisive *f* **supérieure** upper incisor
incontinence *f* incontinence
incontinence *f* **fécale** fecal incontinence
incontinence *f* **urinaire** urinary incontinence

insectifuge

incoordination *f* incoordination
incurvation *f* flexion
indication *f* indication
indications *fpl* thérapeutiques when to use (drugs etc)
indigestion *f* indigestion
inertie *f* utérine uterine inertia
infantilisme *m* genital genital infantilism
infarctus *m* coronary thrombosis
infecté,-e infected
infectieux/infectieuse infectious
infection *f* infection
infection *f* bactérienne bacterial infection
infection *f* cutanée bactérienne mud fever
infection *f* de la glande sébacée ventrale infection of the ventral sebaceous gland
infection *f* de la vessie bladder infection
infection *f* fongique fungal infection
infection *f* virale viral infection
inférieur,-e lower
infertilité *f* infertility
infestation *f* infestation
infestation *f* d'aelurostrangulus abstrusus aelurostrangulus abstrusus infestation
infesté,-e infested
infester infest, to
inflammation *f* inflammation
inflammation *f* de l'uterus inflammation of the uterus
inflammatoire inflammatory
inhabituel/inhabituelle unusual
inhalateur *m* inhaler
inhaler inhale
inhibiteur/ inhibitrice inhibitory
inhibiteur *m* inhibitor
injecté,-e de sang bloodshot
injection *f* injection
injection *f* intradermique intradermic injection
injection *f* intramusculaire intramuscular injection
injection *f* intraveineuse intravenous injection
injection *f* sous-cutanée subcutaneous injection
insecticide *m* insecticide
insectifuge *m* insect repellant

insémination f artificielle artificial insemination
insolation f sunstroke
insomnie f insomnia
insuffisance f insufficiency
insuffisance f cardiaque cardiac insufficiency
insuffisance f hépatique hepatic failure
insuffisance f pulmonaire chronique chronic obstructive pulmonary disease (COPD)
insuffisance f rénale kidney failure
insuline f insulin
intelligent,-e intelligent
interféron interferon
intermission f intermission
intermittent,-e intermittant
internal,-e internal
internal,-e interior
interne internal
intertrigo m intertrigo
intervenir intervene, to
intervention f intervention
intestin m intestine
intestin m grêle small intestine
intestins mpl bowel
intolérance f à intolerance of
intoxication d'aspirine aspirin poisoning
intoxication f alimentaire food poisoning
intoxication f par oxyde de carbone carbon-monoxide poisoning
intramusculaire intramuscular
intranasal,-e intranasal
intraoculaire intraocular
intra-uterin,-e intrauterine
intraveineux/intraveineuse intravenous
intubation f intubation
invagination f invagination
invasif/invasive invasive
involution f involution
iode m iodine
iridocyclite f iridocyclitis
iris m iris
iritis f iritis
irradiation f irradiation

jeûner

irradié,-e irradiated
irrigateur *m* irrigator
irrigation irrigation
irriguer irrigate, to
irritant *m* irritant
irritant,-e irritant
irritation *f* irritation
irritation *f* **des gencives** irritated gums
isolation *f* isolation
isolé,-e isolated
isoler isolate, to
isthme *m* **aortique** aortic isthmus
isthme *m* **de l'utérus** isthmus of the uterus
isthme *m* **thyroïdien** isthmus of the thyroid
ivoire *m* **de la dent** dentine

J

jabot *m* crop
jacobée *f* ragwort
jambe *f* gaskin
jambe *f* leg
jambe *f* lower thigh
japper yelp, to
japper yap, to
jarret *m* hock; hock joint
jarret, pointe *f* **du** point of hock
jarrets *mpl* **clos** cow hocks
jarrets *mpl* **coudés** sickle hocks
jarrets *mpl* **de vache** cow hocks
jaunisse *f* jaundice
javart *m* **cartilagineux** quittor
jeun: à jeun on an empty stomach
jeûne *m* fast
jeûne *m* abstention from food
jeûner fast, to

joint à rotule *m* ball and socket joint
joint *m* joint
joue *f* cheek
jumeau/jumelle twin
jumeaux/jumelles twins
jument *f* mare
jument *f* gestante mare in foal
juste balance *m* right balance

K

kaliémie *f* kalemia
kaolin *m* kaolin
kératine *f* keratin
kératinisation *f* keratinisation
kératite *f* keratitis
kérato-conjonctivite *f* keratoconjunctivitis
kérato-conjonctivite *f* sèche dry keratoconjunctivitis
kératose *f* keratosis
kérion *m* kerion
kinésithérapie *f* physiotherapy
kyste *m* cyst
kyste *m* dermoïde dermoid cyst
kyste *m* graisseux fatty cyst
kyste *m* interdigité interdigital cyst
kyste *m* ovarien ovarian cyst
kyste *m* salivaire salivary cyst
kyste *m* sébacé sebaceous cyst

L

laboratoire *m* pathalogique pathological laboratory (path lab)
labyrinthe *m* ethmoïdal ethmoid(al) labyrinth
labyrinthe *m* olfactif ethmoid(al) labyrinth
lactation *f* lactation
laisse *f* lead

lèvre

lait *m* milk
laminite *f* laminitis
lampe *f* **infrarouge** infrared lamp
lancette *f* lance
langue *f* tongue
laparostomie *f* laparostomy
laparotomie *f* laparotomy
lapereau *m* baby rabbit
lapin *m* rabbit
lapin *m* **nain** dwarf rabbit
lapine *f* female rabbit
larve *f* larva
laryngite *f* laryingitis
laryngospasme *m* laryngospasm
larynx *m* larynx
laurier *m* laurel
laurier *m* **rose** oleander
lavage *m* washing out
lavement *m* enema
lavement *m* **baryté** barium enema
laxatif *m* laxative
laxité *f* laxity
lécher lick, to
leger/legère light
légume *m* vegetable
leishmaniose *f* leishmaniasis
leptospirose *f* leptospirosis
lésion *f* lesion
lésion *f* **cérébrale** brain lesion
lesion *f* **pulmonaire** pulmonary lesion
lésions *fpl* **internes** internal injuries
léthargie *f* lethergy
leucisme *m* leucism
leucocyte *m* leucocyte
leucocytose *f* leucocytosis
leucorrhée *f* leucorrhea
leucose *f* leucosis
leucose *f* **féline** feline leukaemia virus
lèvre *f* lip
lèvre *f* **inférieure** bottom lip
lèvre *f* **supérieure** top lip

libérer unblock, to (intestine etc)
licence *f* permit
licol *m* halter
ligament *m* ligament
ligament *m* **latéral** lateral ligament
ligament *m* **médial** medial ligament
ligament *m* **rotulien** patella ligament
ligament *m* **suspenseur du boulet** suspensory ligament
ligaments *mpl* **croisés** cruciate ligaments
ligature *f* ligature
ligne *f* **blanche** white line
lime *f* **à dents** tooth float blade
lingette *f* **antiseptique** antiseptic wipe
lipome *m* lipoma
liquide *m* **amniotique** amniotic fluid
liquide *m* **antiseptique** antiseptic liquid
liquide *m* **céphalo-rachidien** cerebro-spinal fluid
liquide *m* **synovial** synovial fluid
lisser preen, to
lit *m* bed
lithiase *f* lithiasis
litière *f* cat litter, bedding (horses)
lobe *m* **inférieur** lower lobe (lung)
lobe *m* **moyen** middle lobe (lung)
lobe *m* **supérieur** upper lobe (lung)
longeur *m* length
longévité *f* longevity
longévité *f* life expectancy
lorums *mpl* lore
loucher squint, to
loupe *f* sebaceous cyst
lourd,-e heavy
lupus *m* lupus
luxation *f* **congénitale de la rotule** congenital dislocation of the patella
luxation *f* **de cristallin** lens luxation
luxation *f* **de la rotule** dislocation of the patella
luxation *f* **du globe oculaire** dislocated eyeball
lymphangite *f* lymphangitis
lymphe *f* lymph
lymphocyte *m* lymphocyte

maladie

lymphœdème *m* lymphoedema
lymphosarcomatose *f* lymphosarcomatosis
lymphosarcome *m* lymphosarcoma

M

mâchoire *f* jaw
mâchoire *f* **inférieure** lower jaw
mâchoire *f* **supérieure** upper jaw
magnésium *m* magnesium
maigre underweight
mal *m* **à l'oreille** earache
mal *m* **de l'herbe** grass sickness
mal *m* **de tête** headache
mal *m* **des transports** travel sickness
maladie *f* ill health
maladie *f* sickness
maladie *f* illness
maladie *f* disease
maladie *f* **chronique** chronic disease
maladie *f* **contagieuse** contagious illness
maladie *f* **d'Addison** Addison's disease
maladie *f* **d'Aujeszky** Aujeszky's disease
maladie *f* **de Biermer** pernicious anaemia
maladie *f* **de Carré** canine distemper
maladie *f* **de Cushing** Cushing's disease
maladie *f* **de la graisse jaune** yellow fat disease
maladie *f* **de la queue mouillée** wet tail
maladie *f* **de langeur** wasting disease
maladie *f* **de Ménière** Ménière's disease
maladie *f* **de peau** skin disease
maladie *f* **de Rubarth** Rubarth's disease
maladie *f* **de Scheuermann** Scheuermann's disease
maladie *f* **de Tyzzer** Tyzzer's disease
maladie *f* **du cœur** heart disease
maladie *f* **du foie** liver disease
maladie *f* **hemorragique virale** rabbit haemorraghic disease

maladie f héréditaire hereditary illness
maladie f infectieuse infectious illness
maladie f lysosomale lysosomal disease
maladie f mortelle fatal illness
maladie f naviculaire navicular syndrome
maladie f péridontale dental problem
maladie f pulmonaire pulmonary disease
maladie f rare rare disease
maladie f transmissible infectious disease
maladies fpl cardio-vasculaires cardio-vascular diseases
mâle m male
mâle m furet hob
malformation f cardiaque congénitale congentital heart malformation
malignité f malignancy
malin, maligne malignant
mallassezia m mallassezia
malocclusion f dentaire malocclusion
malpropreté f dirtying
malpropreté f soiling
mamelle f teat
mamelon m nipple
mammite f mastitis
mandibule f mandible
manganèse m manganese
mangeoire f food container
manipulation f manipulation
manipuler handle, to
manque f d'appétit lack of appetite
manque f d'appétit loss of appetite
manque m de lack of
manque m de socialisation poor socialisation
manque m d'exercice lack of exercise
manque m d'hygiène lack of hygiene
manteau m mantle
marasme m marasmus
marcher walk, to
maréchal-ferrant m farrier
marquages m de territoire marking of territory
marquer mark, to
marquer spray, to

métacarpe

mastite *f* mastitis
mastose *f* mastosis
matières *fpl* **grasses** fats
matou *m* tomcat
matrice *f* **unguéale** nail bed
maturité *f* **sexuelle** sexual maturity
mauvaise haleine *f* bad breath
mauvaise santé *f* ill-health
maxillaire maxillary
maxillaire *m* maxilla
maximum maximum
médaille *f* nametag
médecin *m* doctor
médecine *f* medicine
médecine *f* **d'urgence** emergency treatment
médiastin *m* mediastinum
médiastinite *f* mediastinitis
medicament *f* medicine (treatment)
medication *f* medication
médicine *f* **douce** alternative medicine
médicine *f* **douce** complementary medicine
mégacôlon *m* megacolon
mégalooesophage *m* megaoesophagus
mégaoesophage *m* megaoesophagus
mélanine *f* melanin
mélanome *m* melanoma
membrane *f* membrane
membrane *f* **nictatante** nictating membrane
membre *m* **antérieur** fore limb
membre *m* **postérieur** hind limb
méninges *fpl* meninges
méningite *f* meningitis
méningite *f* **externe** pachymeningitis
méningocèle *f* meningocele
menton *m* chin
mérione *m* **de Mongolie** gerbil
mésalliance *f* mismating
mesures *fpl* **préventives** preventative measures
métabolisme *m* metabolism
métacarpe *m* metacarpus
métacarpe *m* pastern

métacarpien/métacarpienne metacarpal
métaplasie *f* metaplasis
métastase *f* metastasis
métatarse *m* metatarsus
métatarse *m* rear pastern
métatarsien/métatarsienne metatarsal
méthode *f* method
métrorragie *f* metrorrhagia
métrorrhée *f* metrorrhea
mettre bas whelp, to
mettre en bas whelp, to
mettre un bandage bandage, to
mettre un pansement sur put a dressing on, to
mettre une sonde à insert a catheter into
miauler mew, to
miauler miaow, to
miction *f* micturition
mieux, meilleur better
millet *m* millet
minimum minimum
mise *f* **en muscle** putting on muscle
mise-bas *f* dropping (a foal)
mises *fpl* **en gardes spéciales** special precautions
mixomatose *f* mixomatosis
mobilité *f* **réduite** reduced mobility
mode *f* **et voie** *f* **d'administration** how to take (drugs etc)
modification *f* modification
moelle *f* **osseuse** bone marrow
molaire *f* molar
monocyte *m* monocyte
monocytose *f* monocytosis
monorchidie *f* monorchidia
montée *f* **de lait** coming-in of milk
mordiller chew, to
mordiller nibble, to
mordre bite, to
morphine *f* morphine
mors *m* bit
mors *m* curb bit
mors *m* **brisé** snaffle
morsure *f* bite

morsure *f* **de serpent (venimeux)** snake bite (poisonous)
morsure *f* **infectée** infected bite
mort *f* **foetale** fœtal death
mort,-e dead
mortel/mortelle fatal
mort-né,-e stillborn
morve *f* equine glanders
mouche *f* fly
moustache *f* moustachial stripe
moustaches *fpl* whiskers
moyen/moyenne average
moyen/moyenne medium
mucocèle *f* mucocele
mucus *m* mucus
mue *f* moulting
muer moult, to
muet/muette mute
muguet *m* thrush
mule *m* mule
muqueuses *fpl* **cyanosées** cyanosed mucus membranes
muscle *m* muscle
muscle *m* **biceps brachial** biceps brachial muscle
muscle *m* **deltoïde** deltoid muscle
muscle *m* **extenseur dorsal du doigt** common digital extensor muscle
muscle *m* **extenseur latéral du doigt** lateral digital extensor muscle
muscle *m* **fessier superficial** superficial gluteal muscle
muscle *m* **fléchisseur médial du doigt** medial head of the deep digital flexor muscle
muscle *m* **fléchisseur superficiel du doigt** superficial digital flexor muscle
muscle *m* **masseter** masseter muscle
muscle *m* **sterno-céphalique** sternocephalicus muscle
museau *m* muzzle
museau *m* **sec** dry nose
muselière *f* muzzle
muserolle *f* noseband
mustang *m* mustang
mutilé,-e mauled
myasthénie *f* myasthenia
myasthénie *f* myasthenia gravis

mycétome *m* mycetoma
mycose *f* mycosis, fungal infection
mycosis *f* **fongoïde** *f* mycosis fungoides
mycotoxicose *f* mycotoxicosis
mycotoxine *f* mycotoxin
mydriase *f* mydriasis
myélite *f* myelitis
myélome *m* myeloma
myélopathie *f* myelopathy
myélopathie *f* **dégénérative** degenerative myelopathy
myglobinurie *f* azoturia
myiase *f* myiasis
myocarde *m* myocardium
myocardite *f* myocarditis
myopathie *f* myopathy
myopie *f* myopia
myopique myopic
myosis *m* miosis
myosite *f* myositis
myotonie *f* myotonia

N

narcolepsie *f* narcolepsy
narcose *f* narcosis
narine *f* nostril
naseau *m* nostril
natrémie *f* natremia
nausée *f* nausea
nécessaire necessary
nécrose *f* necrosis
nécrose *f* **de la cornée** necrosis of the cornea
néonatal,-e neonatal
néoplasie *f* neoplasia
néoplasique neoplastic
néphrite *f* nephritis
néphrose *f* nephrosis
nerf *m* nerve
nerf *m* **optique** optic nerve
nerveux/nerveuse skittish

nerveux/nerveuse highly strung
nervosité *f* excitability
nettoyant *m* **auriculaire** ear cleaning
nettoyer clean, to
nettoyer muck out, to
neurodermatose *f* neurodermatosis
neurologique neurological
neutraliser neutralise, to
neutraliser block, to (pain)
névrite *f* **optique** optic neuritis
nez *m* nose
nez *m* **bouché** blocked nose
niacine *f* niacin
nichoir *m* nestbox
nid *m* nest
niveau *m* **approprié** correct level
nocif/nocive poisonous
nocturne nocturnal
nodule *m* nodule
nœud *m* knot
nœud *m* **sexual** locked/tied mating
noisette *f* hazelnut
noix *m* walnut
nourrir à la main hand rear, to
nourrissant,-e nutritious
noyade *f* drowning
noyer (se) drown, to
nuque *f* neck
nuque *f* poll
nutriment *m* nutriment
nutritif/nutritive nutritious
nutritition *f* nutrition
nyctalopie *f* nyctalopia
nyphomanie *f* nymphomania
nystagmus *m* nystagmus

O

obéissance *f* obedience
obésité *f* obesity
observation *f* observation
observer observe, to
obstruction *f* **de la voie respiratoire** airway obstruction
obstruction *f* **des voies lacrymales** obstructed tear ducts
occasionel/ occasionelle occasional
occiput *m* occiput
occlure occlude, to
occlusion *f* occlusion
occlusion *f* blockage
occlusion *f* **intestinale** obstruction of the intestines
occlusion *f* **intestinale** intestinal blockage
odorat *m* sense of smell
œdème *m* oedema
œdème *m* **aigu du poumon** acute pulmonary oedema
œil m/yeux *mpl* eye/eyes
œillères *fpl* blinkers
œsophage *m* oesophagus
œsophagite *f* oesophagitis
œstrogène *m* oestrogen
œstrus *m* oestrus
œuf *m* egg
oisillon *m* nestling
olécrâne *m* olecranon
olfactif/olfactive olfactory
oligurie *f* oliguria
ombilic *m* umbilicus
ombiliqué,-e umbilical
omnivore omnivorous
omoplate *f* scapula
omoplate *f* shoulder blade
ondulant,-e uneven
ongle *m* talon
ongle *m* claw
ongle *m* nail
onyxis *m* onychitis
opaque opaque
opération *f* operation

ostéochondrose

ophtalmie *f* ophthalmia
ophtalmoscope *m* ophthalmoscope
ophtalmoscopie *f* ophthalmoscopy
oral,-e oral
orchite *f* orchitis
ordonnance *f* prescription
oreille *f* ear
oreille *f* **externe** external ear
oreille *f* **interne** inner ear
oreille *f* **moyenne** middle ear
oreilles *fpl* **poilues** furry ears
oreilles *fpl* **tombantes** dangling ears
oreillette *f* **(du cœur)** auricle
oreillette *f* **droite** right auricle
oreillette *f* **gauche** left auricle
organe *m* organ
orthopédie *f* orthopedics
ortie *f* stinging nettle
os *m* bone
os *m* **accessoire du carpe** accessory carpal bone
os *m* **de la couronne** short pastern bone
os *m* **de seiche** cuttlefish bone
os *m* **du paturon** long pastern bone
os *m* **du pied** pedal bone
os *m* **frontal** frontal bone
os *m* **iliaque** hip bone
os *m* **ilium** ilium
os *m* **lacrimal** lacrimal bone
os *m* **métatarsien principal** large metatarsal bone
os *m* **navicular** navicular bone
os *m* **pénien** penis bone
os *m* **pénien** bacula
os *m* **pubis** pubic bone
os *mpl* **du carpe** carpal bones
os *mpl* **du métatarse** metatarsal bones
oslérose *f* oslerosis
ossature *m* skeletal frame
ostéite *f* osteitis
ostéite *f* **de la troisième phalange** pedalosteitis
ostéochondrite *f* osteochondritis
ostéochondrose *f* osteochondrosis

osteodystrophie f hypertrophique hypertrophic osteodystrophy
ostéofibrose f osteofibrosis
ostéolyse f osteolysis
ostéomyélite f osteomyelitis
ostéopathie f osteopathy
ostéoporose f osteoporosis
osteosarcome m osteosarcoma
otectomie f cutting of the ears
othématome m othematoma
otite f externe ear canker
otite f parasitaire parasitic otitis
otocariose f ear mites
otoscopie f otoscopy
ototoxicité f ototoxicity
ouate f cotton wool
ouate f hydrophile absorbent cotton , cotton wool
ouvrir lance, to
ovaire m ovary
ovariectomie f ovariectomy
ovariectomie f oophorectomy
ovario-hystérectomie f ovariohysterectomy
ovario-hystérectomie f oophorohysterectomy
ovulation f ovulation
ovule m pessary
ovule m ovum
ovuler ovulate
oxygène m oxygen
oxyure m pin worm
oxyuridés mpl equine oxyuris

P

pacemaker m pacemaker
pachyméningite f ossifante pachymeningitis
paille f straw
paître graze, to
palais m fendu cleft palate

palefrenier *m* groom
palper palpate, to
panartérite *f* panarteritis
panarthrite *f* panarthritis
pancréas *m* pancreas
pancréatite *f* pancreatitis
panleucopénie *f* feline panleucopaenia
panniculites *fpl* panniculitis
panophtalmie *f* panophtalmia
pansage *m* **électrique** electric groomer
pansement *m* dressing
pansement *m* **adhésif** adhesive plaster; sticking plaster
panser dress, to (wound etc); put a dressing on, to
panser feed, to (chickens, rabbits)
panser groom, to (horse)
panstéatite *f* pansteatitis
papier *m* **de verre** sandpaper
papier *m* **de verre** glasspaper
papier *m* **déchiqueté** shredded paper
papiers *fpl* **d'identification** identification papers
papillomatose *f* papillomatosis
par voie *f* **orale** by mouth
par voie *f* **rectale** via the rectum
paradonte *m* peridontium
paradontium *m* peridontium
paradontose *f* peridontosis
parage *m* **de la corne** trimming of the hoof
paralyse,-é paralysed
paralysie *f* paralysis
paralysie *f* **faciale** facial paralysis
paraphimosis *m* paraphimosis
paraplégie *f* paraplegia
parasite *m* parasite
parasites *mpl* **intestinaux** intestinal parasites
parasitose *f* parasitosis
parer le sabot trim (hoof), to
parésie *f* paresis
parodontite *f* peridontitis
parodontite *f* periodontal disease
paroi *f* **intestinale** stomach wall
paroi *f* **rectale** rectal wall

paroi *m* wall (stomach etc)
paronychie *f* paronychia
parotiques *fpl* ear coverts
parturition *f* parturition
parvovirose *f* canine parvovirus infection
pas *m* step
pas nécessaire unnecessary
pasteurellose *f* pasteurellosis
patte *f* paw
patte *f* **antérieure** forepaw
patûrage grazing
paturon *m* pastern
paupière *f* eyelid
paupière *f* **inférieure** lower eyelid
paupière *f* **supérieure** upper eyelid
pavillon *m* ear flap
pavillon *m* pinna
payer pay, to
peau *f* skin
peau *f* **désechée** dry skin
peau *f* **morte** scurf
pedigree *m* pedigree
perdre l'appetit lose its appetite, to
peigne *m* **à tirer la crinière** mane pulling comb
peigne *m* **en métal** metal mane comb
pelage *m* coat (of animal)
pellicules *fpl* dandruff
pemphigus *m* pemphigus
pénible difficult
pénis *m* penis
percé,-e punctured
percer lance, to
percher (se) perch, to
perchoir *m* perch
perdre connaissance lose consciousness, to
perdre l'appétit *m* lose one's appetite, to
perforation *f* perforation
perforation *f* **intestinale** intestinal perforation
perfusion *f* **sanguine** blood transfusion
péricarde *m* pericardium
périnatal,-e perinatal

périnée *m* perineum
période *f* **d'incubation** incubation period
périonyxis *m* perionyxis
périople *m* periople
périoste *m* periostium
périostite *f* periostitis
périostose *f* periostosis
péristaltisme *m* peristaltis
péritoine *m* peritoneum
péritonite *f* peritonitis
péritonite *f* **infectieuse féline** feline infectious peritonitis (PIF)
perlèche *f* perleche
perroquet *m* parrot
perruche *f* budgie
perruche *f* budgerigar
perruche *f* **ondulée** parakeet
perspiration *f* perspiration/sweat
perte *f* **d'appétit** loss of appetite
perte *f* **d'auditon** loss of hearing
perte *f* **de connaissance** loss of consciousness
perte *f* **de sang** loss of blood
perte *f* **d'équilibre** loss of balance
perte *f* **des eaux** breaking of the waters
perte *f* **génitale** genital discharge
pertes *fpl* discharge
pertes *fpl* **verdâtres** greenish discharge
peser weigh, to
pessaire *m* pessary
petit gallop *m* canter
petit *m* juvenile
petit sésamoïde *m* distal sesamoid
petit,-e small
petites couvertures *fpl* lesser coverts
petits strongles *mpl* small strongyles
petits strongyles *mpl* small redworms
peur *m* fear
peureux/peureuse timid,frightened
phalange *f* **intermédiaire** middle phalanx
phalange *f* **proximale** proximal phalanx
pharmacie *f* chemist's shop
pharmacie *f* pharmacy

pharmacien *m* **pharmacienne** *f* chemist
pharyngite *f* pharyngitis
pharynx *m* pharynx
phéromone *f* pheromone
phimosis *m* phimosis
phlébite *f* phlebitis
phlegmon *m* phlegmon
phobie *f* phobia
phosphore *m* phosphorus
photophobie *f* photophobia
phtiriose *f* phtirioses
pica *m* pica
picage *m* feather-plucking
pied *m* foot
pied *m* **de pinçard** boxy feet
pieds *mpl* **cagneux** pigeon toes
pieds *mpl* **panards** splay-footed
pierre *f* stone
pierre *f* **à lècher** salt lick
piétinement *m* kneading
piétiner knead, to
pigment *m* pigment
pilule *f* pill
pilule *f* **contraceptive** contraceptive pill
pince *f* toe
pincette *f* tweezers
piqûre de rappel booster injection
piqûre *f* insect bite
piqûre *f* sting
piqûre *f* **d'abeille** bee sting
piqûre *f* **de guêpe** wasp sting
piroplasmose *f* piroplasmosis
pissenlit *m* dandelion
placenta *m* afterbirth
placenta *m* placenta
plaie *f* wound
plaie *f* **de selle** saddle sore
plaie *f* **ulcerée** ulcerated wound
plantaire on the sole of the foot
plante *f* **de pied** sole of the foot
plante *f* **sauvage** wild plant

poitrine

plante *f* **toxique** poisonous plant
plaque *f* **dentaire** dental calculus
plaque *f* **dentaire** dental plaque
plaquettes *fpl* platelets
plasma *m* plasma
plat dans ses arceaux flat-sided
plâtre plaster (for break, fracture)
pleine pregnant
pleine in-foal
plomb *m* lead
plumage *m* plumage
plumage *m* **d'hiver** winter plumage
plumage *m* **nuptial** breeding plumage
plume *f* feather
pneumonie *f* pneumonia
pneumonite *f* **féline** feline pneumanitis
pneumothorax *m* pneumothorax
poche *f* **des eaux** amniotic sac
poids *m* weight
poids *m* **idéal** ideal weight
poignet *m* wrist
poignets *mpl* **étranglés derrière** tied in below the knee
poil: à poil court short-haired
poil: à poil long long-haired
poil: à poil *m* **frisé** rough-haired
poil: à poil *m* **lisse** smooth-haired
poil *m* hair
poil *m* **de couverture** top coat
poils *mpl* **collés** matted fur
pointe *f* **d'aile** wing tip
pointe *f* **de la fesse** point of buttock
pointe *f* **de la hanche** point of hip
pointe *f* **de l'épaule** point of shoulder
pointe *f* **du jarret** hock joint
pointe *f* **du sternum** prosternum
pointe *f* **du sternum** shoulder joint
poison *m* poison
poisson *m* fish
poitrail *m* breast
poitrail *m* chest
poitrine *f* **antérieure** forechest

poitrine *f* **inférieure** chestline
pollakisurie *f* pollakiuria
pollakiurie *f* pollakiuria
polyarthrite *f* polyarthritis
polyarthrite *f* **rheumatoïde** rheumatoid arthritis
polydactylie *f* polydactyly
polydactylisme *m* polydactyly
polydipsie *f* polydipsia
polymyopathie *f* **hypokaliémique** hypokalaemic polymyopathy
polymyosite *f* polymyositis
polype *m* polyp
polyphagie *f* polyphagy
polyurie *f* polyuria
polyuro-polydipsie *f* polyuria-polydipsia
polyvalent,-e general purpose
polyvalent,-e all-purpose
pommade *f* ointment
pommade *f* **antibiotique** antibiotic ointment
pommade *f* **contre les brûlures** burn ointment
pomme *f* apple
pommeau *m* pommel
pompe *f* **stomachale** stomach pump
ponction *f* puncture
ponctionner puncture, to
pondre lay an egg, to
poney *m* pony
poney *m* **de polo** polo pony
Pooper Scooper *m* pooper scooper
portée *f* litter (of kittens etc)
porteur *m* **de germes** germ carrier
posologie *f* posology
posologie *f* dosage
post-cure *f* aftercare
posthite *f* posthitis
postnatal postnatal
posture *f* **anormale** abnormal position
potassium *m* potassium
potomanie *f* potomania
poudre *f* powder
poudre *f* **anti-pouces** flea powder
poulain *m* foal

171

prolapsus

poulain *m* colt
pouliche *f* filly
pouliner foal, to
poulinière *f* brood mare
pouls *m* pulse
poumon *m* lung
poussées *fpl* **dentaires** cutting teeth
poux *mpl* lice
poux *mpl* **de plumes** feather lice
poxvirus *m* poxvirus
précoce early
prèles *fpl* horsetails
prélèvement *m* specimen
prélèvement *m* sample
première phalange *f* phalanx prima
premiers soins *mpl* first-aid
prémolaire *f* premolar
prendre la température take the temperature, to
prendre le mors aux dents take the bit in the teeth, to
préparation *f* **de la couche** preparation for the birth
présentation *f* **antérieure** head presentation
présentation *f* **postérieure** breech presentation
pression *f* **intraoculaire** intraocular pressure
prévenir prevent, to
priapisme *m* priapism
primo-vaccination *f* primary vaccination
prise *f* **de longe** rope burn
prise *f* **de sang** blood sample
procidence *f* procidentia
procidence *f* **de la troisième paupière** procidentia of the third eyelid
proctite *f* proctitis
produit *m* **anti-mouches** fly repellent
produit *m* **antimoustique** mosquito repellent
progestérone *f* progesterone
prognathe prognathic
prognostic *m* prognosis
Programme *m* **de Voyage des Animaux de Compagnie (PVAC)**
    Pet's Passport
prolapsus *m* prolapse
prolapsus *m* **du globe oculaire** prolapse of the eyeball
prolapsus *m* **du rectum** prolapse of the rectum

prolapsus *m* **rectal** rectal prolapse
prolapsus *m* **vaginal** vaginal prolapse
promener (se) à cheval hack to
pronostic *m* prognosis
pro-œstrus *m* pro-oestrus
prophylaxie *f* prophylaxis
propre house-trained
propre clean
propriétaire *m* owner
prostate *m* prostate
prostatectomie *f* prostatectomy
prostatisme *m* prostatism
prostatite *f* prostatitis
protection *f* **territoriale** guarding its territory
protèges-boulets *mpl* fetlock boots
protèges-jarrets *mpl* hock boots
protéine *f* protein
protéinurie *f* proteinuria
prothèse *f* prothesis
prothèse *f* **valvaire** artificial heart valve
prurit *m* pruritis
pseudogestation *f* pseudogestation
pseudotuberculose *f* pseudotuberculosis
psittacose *f* psittacosis
psychodermatoses *fpl* psychodermatoses
psychotrope *m* psychotropic
ptôse *f* ptosis
ptyalisme *m* ptyalism
puberté *f* puberty
puce *f* **électronique** electronic chip
puce *f* **électronique** microchip
puces *fpl* fleas
pulmonaire pulmonary
pulpite *f* pulpitis
pulsation *f* heart beat
pupille *f* pupil
purgatif *m* purgative
purgation *f* purgative
purge *f* purgative
purpura *m* purpura
purulent,-e purulent

pus *m* pus
pyélonéphrite *f* pyelonephritis
pylore *m* pylorus
pyodermite *f* **interdigitée** interdigital pyoderma
pyomètre *m* pyometra
pyorrhée *f* pyorrhea
pyrexie *f* pyrexia
pyurie *f* pyuria

Q

quarantaine *f* quarantine
quartering *m* quartering
quartier *m* quartering
queue *f* tail
queue *f* **grasse** stud tail
queue *f* **tressée** plaited tail

R

rachitisme *m* rickets
radio *f* x-ray
radius *m* radius
rage *f* rabies
raideur *f* stiffness
rainure *f* **vasculaire** vascular groove
ramager warble, to
rasé,-e shaved
raser shave, to
rat *m* rat
rate *f* spleen
râtelier *m* **à fourrage** hay rack
ration *f* serving
raton *m* baby rat
ratte *f* female rat
rayons *mpl* **infrarouge** infrared light

réaction *f* reaction
réadapter readjust, to
réanimation *f* intensive care
réanimation *f* resuscitation
rebondi,-e rounded
rechute *f* relapse
rechuter have a relapse, to
récidivant,-e recurring
récidive *f* recurrence
récidiver recur, to
rectite *f* rectitis
rectrices *fpl* **externes** tail (rectrices)
rectum *m* rectum
reculer back, to
récupérer recover
récupérer recuperate
rééduquer rehabilitate
refroidir cool off
refroidissement *m* chill
régime *m* diet
régime *m* **alimentaire** feeding pattern
régime *m* **végétarien** vegetarian diet
réglementation *f* **d'œstrus** oestrus control
régurgitation *f* regurgitation
régurgiter regurgitate
rein *m* kidney
réinfection *f* re-infection
reins *mpl* loin
relâcher relax
remède *m* cure
rémiges *fpl* **primaires** primaries (feathers)
rémiges *fpl* **secondaires** secondaries (feathers)
rémission *f* abatement (pain, etc)
remplaçant *m* **remplaçante** *f* locum
rénal,-e renal
rendez-vous *m* appointment
renifler sniff, to
renseignements *mpl* information
repos *m* rest
reposer rest, to
reprendre connaissance regain consciousness

reproducteur *m* stud horse
réquinquer (se) perk up, to
résection *f* resection
résection *f* **auriculaire** aural resection
résistance *f* endurance
respiration *f* breathing
respiration *f* respiration
respiration *f* **accélérée** rapid breathing
respiration *f* **artificielle** artificial respiration
respiration *f* **assistée** assisted ventilation
respiration *f* **superficielle** shallow breathing
respirer breathe, to
restes *mpl* left-overs
retard *m* **de croissance** stunted growth
rétention *f* retention
rétention *f* **d'œufs** retention of eggs
rétention *f* **d'urine** retention of urine
rétine *f* retina
rétrécissement *m* stenosis
rhabdomyolyse *f* rhabdomyolysis
rhinite *f* rhinitis
rhinite *f* **chronique** chronic rhinitis
rhinopharyngite *f* rhinopharyngitis
rhino-trachéite *f* **infectieuse féline** feline respiratory disease
     complex
rhododendron *m* rhododendron
rhume *m* cold (illness)
rhume *m* **des foins** hay fever
rigidité *f* **cadavérique** rigor mortis
rincer rinse, to
robe *f* coat (of animal)
robe *f* **d'été** summer coat
robe *f* **d'hiver** winter coat
robe *f* **terne** dull coat
rompu,-e ruptured
ronflement *m* snoring
ronfler snore, to
ronger chew, to
rongeur *m* rodent
ronronner purr, to
rotation *f* **de l'os du pied** pedal bone rotation

rotule *f* patella
rouler (se) roll, to
rupture *f* rupture
rupture *f* **de la poche des eaux** breaking of the waters
rupture *f* **musculaire** muscular rupture
rut *m* mating season
rythme *m* **anormal de cœur** faulty heart rhythm
rythme *m* **cardiaque** heart rate

S

sable *m* sand
sablose *f* feline urological syndrome FUS
sabot *m* hoof
sac *m* **anmiotique** foetal sac
sacrum *m* sacrum
saignement *f* bleeding
saignement *m* **de nez** nosebleed
saigner bleed, to
saillie *f* mating
saillir une jument cover a mare, to
sale dirty
salière *f* supraorbital fossa
salivation *f* **abondante** heavy salivation
salive *f* saliva
salle *f* **d'attente** waiting room
salmonelle *f* salmonella
salmonellose *f* salmonellosis
salpingite *f* salpingitis
s'amaigrir lose weight, to
s'amincir get slimmer, to
sang *m* blood
sangle *f* girth
sans connaisance unconscious
sans papiers unregistered
sarcoïdose *f* sarcoidosis
sarcome *m* **de Kaposi** Kaposi's sarcoma

séquelles

s'atteindre en talon overreach
saturnisme *m* lead poisoning
saturnisme *m* saturnism
saturnisme *m* plumbism
satyriasis *m* satyriasis
sauter jump, to
savon *m* soap
scapulaires *fpl* scapulars
sciatique *f* sciatica
sclérotique *f* sclera
sclérotomie *f* sclerotomy
scrotum *m* scrotum
séborrhée *f* seborrhea
sébum *m* sebum
sécher dry, to
sécheresse *f* des yeux dry eyes
secouer shake, to
secouer la tête shake its head, to
secouer les oreilles shake the ears, to
sédatif *m* sedative
sédation *f* sedation
seime *f* sandcrack
sélenium *m* selenium
selle *f* saddle
sellerie *f* tack
selles *fpl* bowel movement
selles *fpl* stools
selles *fpl* humides watery stools
selles *fpl* malodorantes offensive-smelling stools
selles *fpl* molles soft stools
selles *fpl* sanguinolentes bloody stools
selles *fpl* volumineuses bulky stools
sels *mpl* d'Epsom Epsom salts
semence *f* semen
sénilité *f* senility
sens *m* sense
sensible sensitive
sepsie *f* sepsis
septicémie *f* septicaemia
septique septic
séquelles *fpl* after-effects

seringue *f* syringe
serologie *f* serology
serré,-e de poitrail narrow at the chest
sertolinome *m* Sertoli cell tumeur
sérum *m* serum
sérum *m* antitétanique antitetanus serum
sérum *m* antivenimeux snake bite serum
séton *m* seton
sevrage *m* weaning
sevrer wean, to
sexage *m* sexing
shampooing *m* shampoo
shunt *m* shunt
sialite *f* sialitis
sialogène sialogenous
sialorrhée *f* sialorrhea
sifflement *m* whistling
signe *m* avant-coureur warning sign
signes *mpl* auriculaires signs/indications of ear problems
signes *mpl* de vieillissement signs of ageing
signes *mpl* génitaux signs/indications of genital problems
signes *mpl* nerveux signs/indications of nervousness
signes *mpl* oculaires signs/indications of eye problems
signes *mpl* prémonitoires warning signs
signes *mpl* respiratoires signs/indications of respiratory problems
signes *mpl* urinaires signs/indications of urinary problems
sillon *m* jugulaire jugular groove
s'infecter be infected, to
sinus *m* frontal frontal sinus
sinusite *f* sinusitis
sociable sociable
sodium *m* sodium
soigner look after, to
soins *mpl* d'hygiène hygiene
soins *mpl* quotidiens daily care
soins *mpl* vétérinaires veterinary care
sole *f* sole
sole *f* cornée horny sole
sole *f* sensible sensitive sole
solitaire solitary
solution *f* de stérilisation sterilizing solution

sporadique

sommet *m* **de la tête** crown
somnifère *m* sleeping pill
sondage *m* catheterization
sonde *f* catheter
sonde *f* **d'alimentation** feeding tube
sonde *f* **gastrique** stomach tube
sonde *f* **urétale** urethral catheter
sonder catheterize, to
souffle *m* wind
souffrir be in pain, to
souffrir suffer, to
soumis,-e submissive
soumission *f* submission
sourcil *m* eyebrow
sourd,-e deaf
souriceaux *mpl* young mice
souris *f* mouse
souris *f* **danceuse** dancing mouse
sous-alimentation *f* malnutrition
sous-caudales *fpl* undertail coverts
sous-cutané,-e subcutaneous
sous-gorge *f* throatlash (of bridle)
sous-jacent,-e underlying
sous-poil *m* under coat
sparadrap *m* adhesive plaster
sparadrap *m* sticking plaster
sparadrap *m* **microporeux** micropore tape
spasme *m* spasm
spéculum *m* speculum
sperme *m* sperm
sperme *m* semen
spermogramme *m* sperm analysis
sphincter *m* **anal** anal sphincter
sphincter *m* **pylorique** pyloric sphincter
spina-bifida *m* spinabifida
splénectomie *f* splenectomy
spléneomégalie *f* splenomegaly
spondylite *f* **cervicale** cervical spondylitis
spondylolisthésis *m* spondylolisthesis
spondylopathie *f* spondylopathy
sporadique sporadic

squelette skeleton
stalle *f* stall (horse)
staphylocoque *m* staphylococcus
stéatite *f* steatitis
sténose *f* stenosis
stérile infertile
sterilisateur *m* sterilizer
sternum *m* sternum
steroïde *m* **anabolisant** anabolic steroid
stimulateur *m* **artificiel** pacemaker
stimulateur *m* **cardiaque** pacemaker
stomatite *f* stomatitis
stop *f* stop
strabisme *m* strabismus
streptocoque *m* **béta-hémolytiques** BHS
streptocoques *mpl* streptococci
stress *m* stress
strongyles *fpl* **respiratoires** respiratory strongyles
strongylose *f* **equine** equine strongyloidosis
strongylose *f* **vulgaris** strongyloidosis vulgaris
subaigu/subaiguë subacute
subclinique subclinical
sucre *m* **dans le sang** blood sugar level
suer sweat, to
sueur *f* perspiration/sweat
suffocation *f* suffocation
suffocation *f* choking
sulfamides *mpl* sulphonamides
sulfamidés *mpl* sulphonamides
superficiel,-e superficial
supérieur,-e upper
suppositoire *m* suppository
suppurant,-e supperating
suppuratif/suppurative suppurative
suppuré,-e suppurative
suralimentation *f* overeating
surdité *f* deafness
surdosage *m* overdosage
surdosage *m* excess dose
surdose *f* over dose
surentraînement overtraining

surface *f* **portante** bearing edge
surface *f* **ventrale** ventral surface
surfaix *m* roller; surcingle
suros *mpl* splints (on a horse)
surpoids overweight
surpopulation *f* overpopulation
surveillance *f* monitoring
surveiller monitor, to
sus-caudales *fpl* uppertail coverts
suture *f* suture
suture *f* stitch
suturer stitch, to
symblépharon *m* symblepharon
symptomatique symptomatic
symptôme *f* symptom
syncope *f* syncope
syndrome *m* **d'Horner** Horner's syndrome
syndrome *m* syndrome
syndrome *m* **de Key-Gaskell** Key-Gaskell syndrome
syndrome *m* **éosinophilique félin** feline eosinophilic syndrome
syndrome *m* **immuno-déficitaire acquis** acquired immunity deficiency syndrome
syndrome *m* **vestibulaire** vestibular syndrome
synovie *f* synovial fluid
syringomyélie *f* syringomyelia
système *m* **cardio-vasculaire** cardiovascular system
système *m* **digestif** digestive system
système *m* **immunitaire** immune system
système *m* **lymphatique** lymphatic system
système *m* **nerveux central** central nervous system
système *m* **respiratoire** respiratory system/tract
système *m* **vestibulaire** vestibular system

T

taches *fpl* **noires dans le pelage** black patches in the coat
tachyardie *f* tachycardia

tachypnée *f* tachnypnoea
taille *f* size
tailler les griffes trim the claws, to
talon *m* heel
tampon *m* swab
tapis *m* **caoutchouc** rubber matting
tapis *m* **de garrot** wither pad
tare *f* defect
tare *f* **héréditaire** inborn defect
tarse *m* tarsus
tarsien/tarsienne tarsal
tartre *m* tartar
tatouage *m* tattoo; tattooing
tatouer tattoo, to
taurine *f* taurine
teigne *f* ringworm
teinture *f* tincture
tempérament *m* temperament
tempérament *m* **nerveux** nervous disposition
température *f* temperature
témperature *f* **rectale** rectal temperature
temps *m* time
tendinite *f* tendinitis
tendon *m* tendon
tendon *m* **calcanéen commun** common calcanean tendon
tendon *m* **d'Achille** Achilles tendon
tendon *m* **du fléchisseur profond** deep digital flexor tendon
tendon *m* **du fléchisseur superficiel** common digital flexor tendon
tendon *m* **du perforant** deep digital flexor tendon
tendon *m* **du perforé** common digital flexor tendon
ténesme *m* tenesmus
ténia *m* tapeworm
téniasis *m* teniasis
téno-synovite *f* tenosynovitis
tension *f* blood pressure
tension *f* **intraoculaire** intraocular pressure
tension *f* **oculaire** Intraocular pressure
teratogène teratogenic
terrarium *m* terrarium
test *m* test
test *m* **de Shirmer** Shirmer's test

tester test, to
testicule *m* testicle
testostérone *f* testosterone
tétanie *f* tetany
tétanie *f* **puerpérale** puerperal tetany
tétanos *m* tetanus
tête *f* head
téter feed, to (by the mother)
téter suckle
tétracycline *f* tetracycline
thalamus *m* thalamus
thermomètre *m* thermometer
thermomètre *m* **rectal** rectal thermometer
thiamine *f* thiamin
thorax *m* thorax
thrombocyte *m* platelet
thrombose *f* thrombosis
thrombose *f* **iliaque** iliac thrombosis
thrombus *m* thrombus
thymus *m* thymus
thyroïde *f* thyroid
tibia *m* shinbone
tibia *m* tibia
tic *m* **à l'appui** crib biting
tic *m* **aérophagique** crib biting
tic *m* **de l'ours** weaving
tique *f* tick
tirer pull, to
tissu *m* tissue
tissu *m* **adipeux** adipose tissue
toilettage *m* grooming (dog)
toilette *f* grooming
toilette *f* washing
toison *f* thick coat
toison *f* fleece
tolérance *f* tolerance
tolerance *f* **digestive** easily digested
tomber fall, to
tonique *m* tonic
topique *f* topical
torse *m* torso

torsion *f* torsion
toucher *m* **rectal** rectal examination
touffu,-e bushy
toupet *m* forelock
toupet *m* **tressé** plaited forelock
tour *m* **du canon** cannon's circumference
tourbe *f* peat moss
toux *f* **de chenil** kennel cough
toux *f* **sèche** dry cough
toxémie *f* toxaemia
toxemie *f* **de gestation** toxaemia in pregnancy
toxicodermie *f* toxicoderma
toxidermie *f* toxicoderma
toxine *f* toxin
toxique poisonous
toxocara roundworm
toxoplasma gondii *mpl* toxoplasma gondii
toxoplasmose *f* toxoplasmosis
trachée *f* trachea
trachée *f* windpipe
trachéite *f* tracheitis
tracheobronchite *f* **infectieuse** canine kennel cough
trachéotomie *f* tracheotomy
traîner (se) l'arrière-train scoot to
traitement *m* treatment
traitement *m* **dentaire** dental treatment
traitement *m* **hormonal** hormone treatment
traiter treat, to
tranchant/e sharp
tranquillisant *m* tranquillizer
transmettre (se) transmit, to
transpiration *f* perspiration/sweat
transporter transport, to
transporter take to, to
trauma *m* trauma
travail *m* labour
tremblement *m* tremor
tresse *f* plait, braid
tresser plait, braid, to
trichiasis *m* trichiasis
trichinose *f* trichinosis

ulcère

trichobezoards *mpl* trichobezoards
trichonèmes *mpl* trichonemes
trichure *f* whipworm
tricostéril *m* sterile compress
tripes *fpl* tripe
triscupidite *f* triscupiditis
troène *m* privet
troisième paupière *f* third eyelid
troisième phalange *f* phalanx tertia
trombiculose *f* trombiculosis
trompe *f* **d'Eustache** Eustachian tube
trompe *f* **de Fallope** Fallopian tube
trotter trot, to
troubles *mpl* **de la vue** sight problems
troubles *mpl* **de l'audition** hearing problems
troubles *mpl* **digestifs** digestive problems
truffe *f* nose
truffe *f* **humide** wet nose
truffe *f* **sèche** dry nose
tube *m* **digestif** alimentary canal
tuberculose *f* tuberculosis
tuberosité *f* **du calcanéus** calcanean tuber
tumeur *f* tumour
tumeur *f* **graisseuse** fatty tumour
tumeur *m* **mammaire** mammary tumour
tympan *m* ear drum
typanisme *m* typanism
typhus *m* feline infectious enteritis

U

ulcération *f* ulceration
ulcération *f* **des pattes** ulcerated paws
ulcère *m* ulcer
ulcère *m* **de la cornée** ulcerated cornea
ulcère *m* **de l'estomac** gastric ulcer

ulcère *m* **duodénal** peptic ulcer
ulcéré,-e ulcerated
ulcérer ulcerate, to
urée *f* urea
urémie *f* uraemia
uretère *m* ureter
urgence *f* emergency
urine *f* urine
urine (de cheval) *f* stale
uriner urinate, to; stale, to
urolithiase urolithiasis
urticaire *f* urticaria
usage *m* use
usure *f* **normale** normal wear and tear
utérus *m* uterus
uvéal,-e uveal
uvéite *f* uveitis
uvéite *f* **récidivante** moonblindness

V

vaccin *m* vaccine
vaccin *m* **autogène** autogenous vaccine
vaccin *m* **contra la rage** anti-rabies vaccine
vaccination *f* vaccination
vacciner vaccinate, to
vagin *m* vagina
vaginal,-e vaginal
vaginite *f* vaginitis
vaisseau *m* **capillaire** capillary
vaisseau *m* **éclaté** burst blood vessel
vaisseau *m* **sanguin** blood vessel
valet d'écurie *m* groom
valve *f* **artificielle** artificial heart valve
valvule *f* valve
valvule *f* **triscupide** triscupid valve
vapo *m* atomiser/spray

vétérinaire

vaporisateur *m* atomiser/spray
vaporisateur *m* **anti-puces** flea spray
varicocèle *f* varicocele
variété *f* variety
vascularite *f* vascularitis
vaseline™ *f* vaseline™
veine *f* vein
veine *f* **cave inférieure** vena cava inferioir
veine *f* **cave supérieure** vena cava superioir
veine *f* **coronaire** coronary vein
veine *f* **jugulaire** jugular vein
veine *f* **pulmonaire** pulmonary vein
venin *m* venom
venin *m* poison (snake)
ventilation *f* ventilation
ventre *m* stomach
ventre *m* belly
ventre *m* **de levrette** herring-gutted
ventricule *m* **droit** right ventricle
ventricule *m* **gauche** left ventricle
verdure *f* greenery
vérifier check, to
vermifugation *f* worming
vermifuge *m* worming product
vermifuger worm, to
verrue *f* wart
vers *mpl* worms
vertèbre *f* vertebra
vertèbre *f* **dorsale** dorsal vertebra
vertébre *m* vertebra
vertébré *m* vertebrate
vertèbres *fpl* **caudales** caudal vertebrae
vertèbres *fpl* **caudales/lombaires** lumbar vertebrae
vertébres *fpl* **cervicales** cervical vertebrae
vertébres *fpl* **sacrées** sacral vertebrae
vertèbres *fpl* **thoraciques** thoracic vertebrae
vertige *m* dizziness
vertige *m* vertigo
vésicule *f* **biliaire** gall bladder
vessie *f* bladder
vétérinaire *m* vet/veterinary

vétérinaire *m* **de chevaux** equine veterinarian
viande *f* meat
vidanger empty, to
vidanger drain, to
vieillissement *m* ageing
vieillissement *m* **prématuré** premature ageing
vigueur *f* stamina
villosité *f* villosity
virus *m* virus
visage *m* face
visceral,-e visceral
viscère *m* viscera
viscères *mpl* viscera
vision *f* vision
vitalité *f* vitality
vitaminé,-e vitamin enriched/with added vitamins
vitesse *f* speed
vitesse *f* **de sédimentation globulaire** erythrocyte sedimentation rate
vitesse *f* **de sédimentation sanguine** erythrocyte sedimentation rate
vitiligo *m* vitiligo
voie *f* **respiratoire** airway
voies *fpl* **urinaires** urinary tract
voile *m* **au poumon** shadow on the lung
voler fly, to
volière *f* aviary
vomir vomit, to
vomir be sick, to
vomissement *m* vomiting
vomissements *mpl* **répétés** frequent vomiting
vorace voracious
voûte *f* **du palais** roof of the mouth
voûte *f* **palantine** roof of the mouth
vue *f* **abîmée** deteriorating sight
vulve *f* vulva
vulvite *f* vulvitis

W,X,Y,Z

warfarine *f* warfarin
wheezing *m* wheezing
yearling *m* yearling
yersiniose *f* yersinial infection
yeux *mpl* **globuleux** bulging eyeballs
zinc *m* zinc
zone *f* **auriculaire** ear coverts
zoonose *f* zoonosis
zygote *m* zygote

DOG   CHIEN

1	skull	crâne m
2	cervical vertebrae	vertèbres cervicales fpl
3	dorsal vertebrae	vertèbres dorsales fpl
4	lumbar vertebrae	vertèbres lumbaires fpl
5	sacral vertebrae	vertèbres sacrées fpl
6	coccygeal vertebrae	vertèbres coccygiennes fpl
7	pelvis	bassin m
8	femur	fémur m
9	tibia	tibia m
10	fibula	péroné m
11	tarsus	tarse m
12	metatarsus	métatarse m
13	phalange	phalange f
14	patella	rotule f
15	rib	côte f
16	metacarpus	métacarpe m
17	carpus	carpe m
18	ulna	cubitus m
19	radius	radius m
20	sternum	sternum m
21	humerus	humérus m
22	scapula	scapulaire m

HORSE   CHEVAL

1	skull crâne m
2	atlas atlas m
3	cervical vertebrae vertèbres cervicales fpl
4	dorsal vertebrae vertèbres dorsales fpl
5	lumbar vertebrae vertèbres lumbaires fpl
6	sacral vertebrae vertèbres sacrées fpl
7	coccygeal vertebrae vertèbres coccygiennes fpl
8	femur fémur m
9	fibula péroné m
10	calcaneus calcanéum m
11	metatarsus métatarse m
12	tarsus tarse m
13	tibia tibia m

14	patella rotule f
15	pelvis bassin m
16	rib côte f
17	sternum sternum m
18	ulna cubitus m
19	proximal sesamoid grande sésamoïde m
20	distal sesamoid petit sésamoïde m
21	phalange phalange f
22	metacarpus métacarpe m
23	carpus carpe m
24	radius radius m
25	humerus humérus m
26	scapula scapulaire m

192

CAT   CHAT

PAW   PATTE

1	nose leather	truffe *f*
	whiskers	moustaches *f pl*
3	nictitating membrane	paupière *f* interne
4	lower eyelid	paupière *f* inférieure
5	upper eyelid	paupière *f* supérieure
6	ear	oreille *f*
7	eyelashes	cils *m*
8	pupil	pupille *f*
9	muzzle	museau *m*
10	back	dos *m*
11	tail	queue *f*
12	paw	patte *f*
13	fur	fourrure *f*

1B	claw	griffe *f*
	pad	coussinet *m*
2B	digital pad	coussinet *m* digité
3B	palmar pad	coussinet *m* palmaire
4B	carpal pad	coussinet *m* carpien
5B	dew pad	coussinet *m* de l'ergot
6B	dew claw	ergot *m*

BIRD   OISEAU

1	lower mandible / mandibule *f*
2	upper mandible / maxillaire *m* supérieur
3	nostril / narine *f*
4	lore / lorum *m*
5	forehead / front *m*
6	crown / calotte *f*
7	eye ring / anneau *m* oculaire
8	eyebrow stripe / raie *f* sourcillière
9	auriculars / région *f* auriculaire
10	nape / nuque *f*
11	back / dos *m*
12	wing covert / tectrice *f* sus-alaire
13	rump / croupion *m*
14	tail feather / rectrice *f*
15	upper tail covert / tectrice *f* sus-caudale
16	under tail covert / tectrice *f* sous-caudale
17	wing / aile *f*
18	claw / griffe *f*
19	tarsus / tarse *m*
20	hind toe / doigt *m* postérieur
21	foot / patte *f*
22	outer toe / doigt *m* externe
23	middle toe / doigt *m* médian
24	inner toe / doigt *m* interne
25	thigh / cuisse *f*
26	abdomen / abdomen *m*
27	flank / flanc *m*
28	breast / poitrine *f*
29	throat / gorge *f*
30	malar region / région *f* malaire
31	chin / menton *m*

194

DOG BREEDS
LES RACES DE CHIENS

Affenpinscher	Affenpinscher *m*
Afghan Hound	Lévrier Afghan *m*
Airedale Terrier	Terrier Airedale *m*
Akita Inu	Akita *m*
Alaskan Malamute	Malamute *m* d'Alaska
American Cocker Spaniel	Epagneul *m*Américain
American Foxhound	Fox-Hound *m*Américain
American Staffordshire Bull Terrier	Terrier Staffordshire Américain *m*
Australian Silky Terrier	Terrier Silky *m*
Australian Terrier	Terrier Australien *m*
Basenji	Basenji *m*
Basset Hound	Basset *m*
Beagle	Beagle *m*
Beauceron	Berger de Beauce ou Beauceron *m*
Bedlington Terrier	Terrier Bedlington *m*
Belgian Shepherd Dog	Berger Belge *m*
Bernese Mountain Dog	Chien de Montagne Bernois *m*
Bichon Frise	Bichon Frisé *m*
Black and Tan Coon Hound	Coonhound *m* Noir et Fauve *m*
Bloodhound	Limier *m*
Border Terrier	Border Terrier *m*
Borzoi	Barzoï *m*
Boston Terrier	Terrier de Boston *m*
Bouvier des Flandres	Bouvier des Flandres *m*
Boxer	Boxer *m*
Breton Spaniel	Épagneul *m* Breton
Briard	Briard *m*

Bull Terrier	Bull Terrier *m*
Bulldog	Bulldog *m*; Bouledogue *m*
Bullmastiff	Bullmastiff *m*
Cairn Terrier	Cairn *m*
Cardigan Welsh Corgi	Corgi *m* Cardigan Gallois
Chesapeake Bay Retriever	Chesapeake *m*
Chihuahua	Chihuahua *m*
Chinese Crested	Crested Chinois *m*
Chow Chow	Chow Chow *m*
Cocker Spaniel	Cocker *m*
Cocker Spaniel (English)	Épagneul *m* Cocker Anglais
Collie	Colley *m*
Curly Coated Retriever	Retriever *m* Bouclé
Dachshound	Teckel *m*
Dalmatian	Dalmatien *m*
Dandie Dinmont Terrier	Dandie Dinmont *m*
Dobermann	Doberman Pinscher *m*
Elkhound	Elkhound *m* Norvégien
English Foxhound	Fox-hound *m* Anglais
English Setter	Setter *m* Anglais
English Springer Spaniel	Épagneul *m* Springer Anglais
Field Spaniel	Field Spaniel *m*
Finnish Spitz	Loulou Finlandais *m*
Flat Coated Retriever	Flat-Coated Retriever *m*
French Bulldog	Bulldog Français *m*
French Spaniel	Épagneul *m* Français
German Shepherd Dog	Berger Allemand *m*
German Short-haired Pointer	Pointer Allemand à poils ras *m*
German Wire-haired Pointer	Pointer *m* Allemand à poils durs
Golden Retriever	Golden Retriever *m*
Gordon Setter	Setter Gordon *m*
Great Dane	Danois *m*

Greyhound	Lévrier *m*
Griffon Bruxellois	Griffon Bruxellois *m*
Groenenendael (Belgian Shepherd Dog)	Groenendael *m*
Harrier	Harrier *m*
Hungarian Kuvasz	Kuvasz *m*
Hungarian Puli	Puli *m*
Hungarian Vizsla	Vizsla *m*
I haven't the faintest idea!!	Nizinny *m*
Ibizan Hound	Ibizan Hound *m*
Irish Setter	Setter Irlandais *m*
Irish Terrier	Terrier Irlandais *m*
Irish Water Spaniel	Épagneul *m* Irlandais
Irish Wolfhound	Chien Loup Irlandais *m*
Italian Greyhound	Petit Lévrier Italien *m*
Japanese Chin	Chin ou Epagneul Japonais *m*
Keeshond	Keeshond *m*
Kerry Blue Terrier	Terrier Kerry Blue *m*
King Charles Spaniel	Épagneul *m* du Roi Charles
Komondor	Komondor *m*
Labrador Retriever	Labrador *m*
Lakeland Terrier	Lakeland Terrier *m*
Lhasa Apso	Lhasa Apso *m*
Maltese Terrier	Bichon Maltais *m*
Manchester Terrier	Manchester Terrier *m*
Mastiff	Mastiff *m*
Miniature Bull Terrier	Petit Bull Terrier *m*
Miniature Pinscher	Pinscher Miniature *m*
Newfoundland	Terre-Neuve *m*
Norfolk Terrier	Terrier Norfolk *m*
Norwich Terrier	Terrier Norwich *m*
Old English Sheepdog or Bobtail	Berger Anglais ou Bobtail *m*

Papillon	Papillon *m*
Pekinese	Pékinoi *m*
Pembroke Welsh Corgi	Corgi Pembroke Gallois *m*
Petit Basset Griffon Vendeen	Petit Basset Griffon Vendéen *m*
Pharoah Hound	Chien des Pharaons *m*
Pointer	Pointer *m*
Pomeranian	Loulou *m* de Poméranie
Poodle	Caniche *m*
Portugese Water Dog	Water Dog Portugais *m*
Pug	Pug *m*
Pyrenean Mountain Dog	Berger *m* des Pyrénées
Pyrenean Mountain Dog	Montagne des Pyrénées *m*
Rhodesian Ridgeback	Ridgeback *m* de Rhodésie
Rottweiler	Rottweiler *m*
Rough Collie	Colley *m* à poils longs
Rough-coated Griffon Bruxellois	Griffon *m* à poils drus
Saluki	Saluki *m*
Samoyed	Samoyed *m*
Schipperke	Schipperke *m*
Scottish Deerhound	Limier Ecossais *m*
Scottish Terrier	Terrier Ecossais *m*
Sealyham Terrier	Terrier Sealyham *m*
Shar-Pei	Shar-Pei *m*
Shetland Sheepdog	Berger des Shetland *m*
Shih Tzu	Shih Tzu *m*
Siberian Husky	Huskie *m*
Skye Terrier	Skye Terrier *m*
Smooth-haired Fox Terrier	Fox Terrier *m* à poils lisses
Soft-coated Wheaten Terrier	Wheaten Terrier *m*
St. Bernard	Saint-Bernard *m*
Schnauzer	Schnauzer *m*

Schnauzer, Giant	Schnauzer *m* Géant
Schnauzer, Miniature	Schnauzer *m* Nain
Schnauzer, Standard	Schnauzer *m* Moyen
Staffordshire Bull Terrier	Bull Terrier Staffordshire *m*
Sussex Spaniel	Épagneul *m* du Sussex
Tervueren (Belgian Shepherd Dog)	Tervuren Belge *m*
Tibetan Spaniel	Épagneul *m* Tibétain
Tibetan Terrier	Terrier Tibétain *m*
Weimaraner	Weimaraner *m*
Welsh Springer Spaniel	Épagneul *m* Gallois
Welsh Terrier	Terrier Gallois *m*
West Highland White Terrier	Westie *m*
Whippet	Whippet *m*
Wire-haired Fox Terrier	Fox Terrier *m* à poils durs
Yorkshire Terrier	Terrier Yorkshire *m*

CAT BREEDS
LES RACES DE CHATS

Abyssinian	Abyssin *m*
Abyssinian Blue	Abyssin Bleu *m*
American Curl	Américain Curl *m*
American Shorthair	Américain *m* à poil court
American Wirehair	Américain *m* à poil dur
Balinese	Balinais *m*
Bengal	Bengal *m*
Birman	Birman *m*
Bombay	Bombay *m*
Burmese	Burmèse *m*
California Spangled Cat	California Spangled *m*
Chartreux	Chartreux *m*
Cornish Rex	Rex de Cornouailles *m*
Cymric	Cymric *m*
Devon Rex	Rex du Devon *m*
English Shorthair	Anglais *m* à poil court
Egyptian *m* Mau	Mau Egyptien *m*
European	Européen/Européenne
Exotic Shorthair	Exotique *m* à poil court
Havana Brown	Havana Brown *m*
Herman	Herman *m*
Himalayan	Himalayen *m*
Japanese Bobtail	Bobtail *m* japonais
Korat	Korat *m*
Maine Coon	Maine Coon *m*
Manx	Manx *m* ; chat de l'ile de Man
Norwegian Forest cat	Chat *m* des Bois de Norvège
Ocicat	Ocicat *m*

Ojos Azules	Ojos Azules *m*
Oriental Shorthair	Oriental *m* à poil court
Persian	Persan *m*
Ragdoll	Ragdoll *m*
Rex	Rex *m*
Russian Blue	Bleu *m* de Russie
Scottish Fold	Scottish Fold *m*
Selkirk Rex	Selkirk Rex *m*
Siamese	Siamois *m*
Siberian	Sibérien *m*; Chat *m* de Sibérie
Singapore; Singapura	Chat *m* de Singapour
Snowshoe	Snowshoe *m*
Somali	Somali *m*
Sphynx	Sphynx *m*
Tonkinese	Tonkinois *m*
Turkish Angora	Angora Turc *m*
Turkish Van	Turc du lac de Van *m*

HORSE BREEDS
LES RACES DE CHEVAUX

Andalusian	Andalou *m*
Appaloosa	Appaloosa *m*
Arab	Arabe, le cheval
Ardennes horse	Ardennais, le cheval
Belgian trotter	Trotteur belge *m*
Boulonnais	Boulonnais *m*
Breton	Breton, le cheval
Camargue	Camarguais, le cheval
Connemara	Connemara, le poney
English Thoroughbred	Pur-Sang Anglais *m*
French trotter	Trotteur francais *m*
Friesian	Frison, le cheval
Hafflinger Pony	Hafflinger *m*
Highland pony	Highland, le poney
Icelandic pony	Islandais, le poney
Lipizzaner	Lipizan *m*
Lusitano	Lusitanien, le cheval
New Forest pony	New Forest, le poney
Palomino	Palomino *m*
Percheron	Percheron *m*
Quarter Horse	Quarter Horse *m*
Selle Français; French Saddle-Horse	Selle Français *m*
Shetland pony	Shetland, le poney
Welsh pony; Welsh cob	Welsh poney *m*; Welsh cob *m*

Note: None of the above Breed Lists are comprehensive

HADLEY PAGER INFO PUBLICATIONS

All publications listed are French-English and English-French

CONCISE DICTIONARY OF HOUSE BUILDING (Arranged by Trades)

Paperback, 2005 Third Edition, 304 pages, 210 x 144 mm
ISBN 1-872739-11-3   Price: £27.00

- Dictionary is divided into 14 sections covering the various stages and trades employed in house building: Architect, Earthworks and Foundations, Builder, Carpenter and Joiner, Woods and Veneers, Roofer, Ironmonger, Metals, Plumber, Glazier, Electrician, Plasterer, Painter and Decorator, Colours.
- Over 10.000 terms in each language. The book is the ideal companion when liaising with tradespeople or when visiting builders' merchants and DIY stores

GLOSSARY OF HOUSE PURCHASE AND RENOVATION TERMS

Paperback, 2000, Fourth Edition, 56 pages, 210 x 148 mm
ISBN 1-872739-08-3   Price: £7.50

- Provides over 2000 French words and phrases used by estate agents, notaires, mortgage lenders, builders, decorators, etc.

GLOSSARY OF FRENCH LEGAL TERMS

Paperback, 1999, 114 pages, 210 x 148 mm
ISBN 1-872739-07-5   Price: £12.00

- Provides over 4000 French legal words and phrases associated with legislation falling within the Civil Code and the Penal Code, (eg house purchase and wills), but company and commercial legislation is not covered.

GLOSSARY OF GARDENING AND HORTICULTURAL TERMS

Paperback, 2004, Third Edition, 72 pages, 210 x 148 mm
ISBN 1-872739-14-8   Price: £8.50

- The glossary includes nearly 2000 gardening and horticultural terms
- The glossary matches up the familiar French and English names of pot and garden flowering plants and shrubs which are not readily available elsewhere.

CONVERSATIONAL FRENCH MADE EASY
By Monique Jackman

Paperback 2005 256 pages, 210 x 145 mm
ISBN 1-872739-15-6   Price £9.95

- Ideal for those with a basic knowledge of French who wish to improve and enhance their conversational skills. Particularly useful for those who have recently moved to France or have a second home there
- The book covers some 120 French verbs with more than one meaning in French. The parallel French and English translations make working alone possible, or in pairs or groups of.family members and friends

HADLEY PAGER INFO PUBLICATIONS

HADLEY'S CONVERSATIONAL FRENCH PHRASE BOOK

Paperback, 1997, 256 pages, 148 x 105 mm
ISBN 1-872739-05-9   Price: £6.00
- Over 2000 French/English phrases and 2000 English/French phrases
- Eleven conversational topic vocabularies
- Aide-memoire key word dictionary

HADLEY'S FRENCH MOTORING PHRASE BOOK & DICTIONARY

Paperback, 2001, 176 pages, 148 x 105 mm
ISBN 1-872739-09-1   Price: £6.00
- Asking the Way, Road Signs, Car Hire, Parking, Breakdowns, Accidents, Types of
- Vehicle, Cycling and Motor Sports. Extensive Dictionary
- Over 3000 words and phrases included

GLOSSARY OF MEDICAL, HEALTH AND PHARMACY TERMS

Paperback, 2003, First Edition, 203 pages, 210 x 148 mm
ISBN 1-872739-12-1   Price: £12.50
- Provides over 3000 medical, health and pharmacy terms, including common illnesses and diseases, anatomical, first-aid and hospital terms. Brief aide-memoire definitions
- Pharmacy terms include medicines, toiletries, cosmetics, health and pharmaceuticals

HADLEY'S FRENCH MEDICAL PHRASE BOOK

By Susan Kirkham and Alan Lindsey
Paperback. 2004, 156 pages, 148 x 105 mm
ISBN 1-872739-13-X   Price £6.00

- Invaluable to travellers in France or in the UK seeking medical advice or medical treatment   Topics included are At the Doctor's, At the Hospital, Baby's, Children's, Young People's, Male and Female Health. Also At the Chemist's, At the Dentisi, At the Optician's, Accidents and •Emergencies.
- A Reference section is also included

Hadley Pager publications are available through good booksellers or can be obtained directly
from Hadley Pager Info by sending a cheque to cover the price
(postage is free within the UK, add 10% if outside the UK)
to **Hadley Pager Info, PO Box 249, Leatherhead, KT23 3WX, England**.

Web Site: http://www.hadleypager.com
Latest Publication List available on request.   Email: hpinfo@aol.com